A MEDICAL MISCELLANY

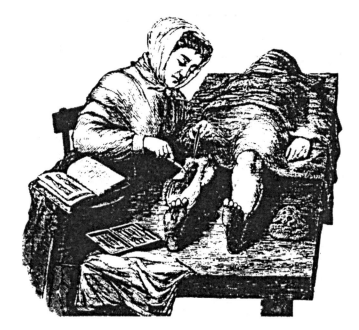

FOR GENEALOGISTS

Dr. Jeanette L. Jerger

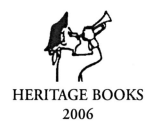

HERITAGE BOOKS
2006

HERITAGE BOOKS

AN IMPRINT OF HERITAGE BOOKS, INC.

Books, CDs, and more—Worldwide

For our listing of thousands of titles see our website
at
www.HeritageBooks.com

Published 2006 by
HERITAGE BOOKS, INC.
Publishing Division
65 East Main Street
Westminster, Maryland 21157-5026

Other books by the author:

Old Soldiers' Home: A History and Necrology of the Northwestern Branch, National Home for Disabled Volunteer Soldiers, Wauwatosa, Wisconsin, 1864-1900

International Standard Book Number: 978-0-7884-0375-3

Table of Contents

Preface

Over time, research in genealogy has led me along many paths of discovery. A particular discovery has sent me on a journey that has been exciting and enlightening and, very likely, never ending. I found a notation on my great-grandfather's Civil War pension application stating that his inability to work was due to being "salivated" during his time in service. Although I have a strong background in medical knowledge, I was unable to find a contextual understanding of "salivated" in current medical resources. By exploring old medical resources, I finally did learn the meaning of 'salivated.' That's when I came up with the idea for this book in which I could list other difficult and obscure medical terms relevant to the work of genealogists.

My exploration of old medical resources provided basic information regarding mainstream medical understanding in times past. I also sought other resources to firm up understanding from points of view outside the mainstream, that is, variations in cultures and beliefs as they related to cause, prevention, and treatment of disease. I did not overlook myth and magic as they weave in and out of the healing arts.

Generally, I selected items for this collection based on the frequency with which they are found in the literature and for their representation of historical medical concepts. I added time frames whenever I could confirm them in at least two sources. Most often origins were hazy, and through the centuries use diminished but never quite vanished. I have blended lay terminology and medical terminology to clarify medical concepts for the general reader.

Items in this collection consist of medical descriptions reflecting 19th century understanding of the most prevalent diseases; definitions of obsolete or infrequently used terms that assist in contextual understanding; popular herbal remedies; treatments for prevention and cure of disease; ethnic variations in cause, prevention, and treatment of disease; and historical reference points.

v

I hope that the information found herein will not only provide the reader with a greater understanding of the healing arts of the past but that it also provides a flavor of life in the time of our forebears.

Dr. Jeanette L. Jerger
September, 1995

Guide for Use

* The *Miscellany* is set up in alphabetical order.

* It is cross-referenced to help direct the reader to find information quickly. For example, if information were needed about "ship fever": under **"SHIP FEVER"** there is found the phrase "Also typhus." Go to **"TYPHUS"** and you will find the other names that the disease is known by and a description of the disease.

* Obscure or obsolete terms, including some recurring, non-medical terms, used in the definitions can be found in the *Miscellany*. For example, the term "regulars" is noted in the description of an item. Look up **REGULARS** and you will find the definition. Or the word "antiquity" appears in several definitions. Look up **ANTIQUITY** and you will find a definition.

* A few items required several definitions. Each definition is found under the item and is separated from other definitions in a new paragraph and by using the conjunction "And" to begin the sentence. For example:
  APOPLEXY
  The condition resulting from hemorrhage or plugging of a blood vessel in the brain or spinal cord.
  And the bursting of a blood vessel in another organ, such, as the lungs or liver.

* Variations in grammatical form and/or spelling of certain terms have been placed in brackets following the term. For example:
  BUBOES [BUBO, BUBOS]

* Variant spellings that arose from pronunciation, e.g. "ager" from "ague," are listed as separate entries.

* References used to compile the data are found in the back of the book for those who wish to do further research in this area.

A Medical Miscellany for Genealogists

ABDOMINAL DROPSY
Also hydrops ascites. An abnormal collection of fluid in the abdominal cavity.

ABDOMINAL TYPHUS
Also typhoid fever.

ABRAHAM MEN
Beggars who pretended to be insane or sick as a means to gain the sympathy of potential givers. The name came from a ward of Bedlam, a hospital for the insane in England. In the 17th century, men from this ward were sent out to beg as a routine part of their stay at the hospital.

ABUNDANCE
Also uberty. The ability to conceive and bear children.

ACACIA
Also gum arabic.

ACNE ROSACEA
Also bottle nose.

ACTIVE IMMUNIZATION
Also immunization.

ACUPUNCTURE
A treatment first used in ancient China for the relief of pain and the treatment of disease. It is believed that by inserting fine needles into selected areas of the skin opposite powers in the body, Yin and

Yang, could be brought into balance thereby controlling pain and/or healing disease.

ACUTE DISEASE
An illness characterized by a rapid onset, a short course, and pronounced symptoms.

ADAM'S APPLE
Also pomum adami, prominentia laryngea. The prominence on the throat formed by the underlying thyroid cartilage very evident in the male. Once believed to be caused by the forbidden apple caught in Adam's throat.

ADEPS
Also lard.

AFFECTION
Disease.

AFRICAN AMERICAN HEAD LOUSE REMEDY
Also head louse remedy.

AFRICAN AMERICAN TOOTH CARE
Also tooth care.

AFRICAN BLACK MAGIC
The work of the sorcerer. It was believed that they cast spells in cemeteries to cause clients' enemies sickness or death, they made medicine and charms to work evil on others, and they raised zombies to carry out their work. See **SORCERY.**

AFRICAN PRIEST
A cult leader who generally worked for good by countering black magic. The African Priest used special charms and herbal medicines to divert evil. See **WHITE MAGIC.**

AGER
Also ague.

AGONAL THROMBOSIS
Also agony clot.

AGONY

Also death struggle. Involuntary body movements occurring just before death. Prior to the 20th century, believed to be caused by severe pain and/or an unwillingness to die.

AGONY CLOT

A semisolid mass of blood believed, until the 20th century, to be formed in the heart during the act of dying in individuals with a history of heart failure. Characterized by severe pain about the heart and a sense of impending death.

AGUE

Also malaria.

And a generic term used for any illness characterized by episodes of chills, fever, and sweating.

AGUE CAKE

A chronic enlargement of the spleen noted in association with chills, fever and pain under the lower left rib.

AGUE TREE

Also sassafras tree.

ALBINISM

A congenital condition characterized by white skin, light-colored hair, and pink eyes. It is due to the absence of pigment, the normal coloring matter of the body.

ALBINO

A person with albinism.

And a "white" descendant of "black" parents.

ALBUMINURIA

Also Bright's disease.

ALCHEMY

A primitive scientific system based on occult ideas of perfection and purification, ancient astrology, and chemical experimentation. Its chief concerns

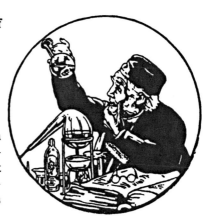

were with changing base metals into gold and finding a universal remedy for disease. It was known to have existed in the 4th century and was widely practiced from the 13th to the 17th centuries.

ALCOHOLIC CEREBRAL EDEMA
Also wet brain.

ALIENIST
Also psychiatrist. A medical specialist in mental diseases.

ALKERMES
A cordial used to treat melancholy in the 16th and 17th centuries. It was made up of cider, rose water, sugar flavoring, and a red coloring agent made of the dried bodies of kermes insects.

ALLOPATHY
A system of disease treatment using remedies that produce effects different from the disease being treated. The term was created by Dr. Samuel Hahnemann, the founder of homeopathy, in an effort to distinguish between homeopathic practice and the practice of the "regulars." The label was not accepted by the regulars, although, at times, their practice was allopathic, such as when sedatives were used to treat an excited state. Compare **HOMEOPATHY.**

ALMS HOUSE
Also poorhouse. A home supported by the community for the sickly, the elderly, the poor and those unable to care for themselves.

ALOE
A plant native to Africa used as a healing herb since antiquity. The juice has been used in folk medicine throughout the world for multiple conditions including skin disorders, breathing problems and constipation.

ALTERATIVE [ALTERANT]
A remedy derived from animal, vegetable or mineral that was believed to correct the processes of nutrition and repair body organs and body systems. Popular alteratives during the 19th century were arsenic, iodine, and mercury. Herbs, such as camomile, and oils from the livers of fish, such as cod, were included in this classification.

ALYON'S OINTMENT
A salve prepared with lard and nitric acid commonly used by the "regulars" until the late 19th century to treat skin diseases.

AMATIVENESS
Sexual and social impulses.

AMAUROSIS
Blindness without evidence of disease in the eye itself.

AMBER
The fossil resin of pine cones. It was given orally for hysteria, whooping cough, and menstrual problems, and applied locally to the skin for chronic rheumatism, whooping cough and infantile convulsions until the early 20th century. Amber necklaces were placed on infants to ward off illnesses.

AMBERGRIS [AMBERGREASE]
A substance taken from the sperm whale's intestine that was used as a remedy for chronic catarrh, low fevers, and hysteria in the 19th century. It was later used as a perfume.

AMERICAN MANDRAKE
Also May apple.

AMERICAN PLAGUE
Also yellow fever.

AMMONIA WATER
Also hartshorn.

AMULET
A gem, or other object, carried about the person to ward off evil.

ANAL PROLAPSE
Also falling of the fundament.

ANCIENT HISTORY
Also antiquity.

ANCYLOSTOMIASIS [ANCHYLOSTOMIASIS, ANKYLOSTOMIASIS]
Also hookworm disease.

ANEMIA
Also poverty of the blood. A deficiency in the quantity or quality of the blood, anemia could be local or general. A local anemia was caused by obstruction of the blood supply to a part of the body. (The phrase "local anemia" fell into disuse in the mid-1900s and was replaced by the term "ischemia.") General anemia was caused by wasting diseases and severe blood loss.

ANGEL MAN
An African priest whose traditional religious beliefs had been influenced by Christianity and Islam in the mid-1800s. Visions of angels became part of their ritual of communing with the spirits of the dead. Their healing methods included immersing the sick in sacred rivers. In the late 1800s they added prophecy to their role.

ANGEL'S TRUMPET
Also jimsonweed.

ANGINA
Any inflammatory disease of the throat.
And any severe cramp-like pain.

ANIMAL MAGNETISM
Also braidism, hypnotism, mesmerism, trance. A method of treating illness developed by Dr. Franz Mesmer in the late 1700s. He believed that there was a magnetic fluid, a force, in the body of the healer by means of which ailments of others could be cured. He used that force to place the patient in a condition resembling sleep, during which the patient received suggestions from the healer. After the sleep ended, the patient would follow the suggestions. Dr. Mesmer's method was the forerunner of what was later to be known as hypnosis.

ANODYNE
A remedy that gives relief from pain.

ANTEBELLUM
The period of time prior to the Civil War.

ANTHRAX
Also splenic fever, woolsorter's disease. An acute infectious

disease of cattle and sheep that can be transmitted to humans characterized by boils on the skin and inflammation of the lungs, pleura, and mucous membranes of the intestine. The term "carbuncle" was first used to denote this condition but fell into disuse in the 19th century.

ANTIPERIODIC
A generic term for a remedy used to prevent the regular recurrence of a disease or a symptom. Specifically, an antimalarial remedy.

ANTIPHLOGISTIC
A generic term for a remedy used to counteract inflammation and fever.

ANTIQUITY
Also ancient history. The period of time before the end of the Western Roman Empire, circa 476 A.D.

ANTISEPTIC
Also germicide.

APERIENT
A mild laxative.

APIUM
Also celery seed. An herbal remedy used as a sedative and a tonic.

APOPLECTIC FIT
Also apoplexia, stroke. A sudden change in level of consciousness and a loss of control of body movement caused by hemorrhaging within the cranial cavity.

APOPLEXIA
Also apoplectic fit.
And also apoplexy.

APOPLEXY
Also apoplexia. A condition resulting from an apoplectic fit characterized by paralysis or limitation in the ability to control body movements, with or without loss of consciousness, and often leaving

the affected individual in a chronic state of debilitation.

And the bursting of a blood vessel in another organ, such as the lungs or liver.

APOTHECARY

Originally a shopkeeper, a grocer, who dealt with a specialized product. In 19th century England and Ireland the apothecary became a licensed practitioner who prescribed and dispensed drugs after 6 to 12 months of educational preparation. In colonial America the apothecary dispensed remedies and practiced medicine "irregularly."

APOTROPAIC

Constructed to protect one from evil.

APPLE OF THE EYE

Also eyeball. The globe shaped body found in the eye socket.

ARDENT FEVER

Any illness characterized by very high fevers.

ARDENT SPIRITS

Any alcoholic drink.

ASAFETIDA [ASAFOETIDA, ASSAFETIDA, ASSAFOETIDA]

A thick gum obtained from the root of a plant native to Asia. This plant is believed to have been brought to Europe from Arabia in the 2nd century. Prior to the 20th century, it was used to treat hysteria, respiratory affections, and tympanites. The strong garlic-like odor of the gum was believed to contribute to the cure of the hysterical patient. It was worn in a small bag around one's neck as an amulet to ward off disease. It continues to be used as a condiment.

ASIATIC CHOLERA

Also cholera.

ASTHMA

Also epilepsy of the lung. A condition known since antiquity. A term first used to indicate any breathing difficulty, especially if experienced in a horizontal position. Many herbal remedies were prescribed for this condition. In the 19th century the condition was further defined to be a bronchial tube condition characterized by difficulty breathing, a cough, and a feeling of suffocation. It was believed to be a neurosis.

ASTRINGENT

A medicine which constricts living tissue causing the constriction of blood vessels and thereby arresting discharge from the tissue.

AUTUMNAL CATARRH

Also cow cold, hay asthma, hay fever, horse cold, miller's asthma, rose cold, snow cold. An acute irritating inflammation of the mucous membranes of the eyes and breathing passages along with itching, sneezing, and great watery discharge. An asthmatic attack was considered to be a common symptom. Until the early 1900s, it was believed to be due to diseased conditions of the nose and/or the pollen of grasses.

BACKACHE

Also lumbago.

BACKHOUSE

Also privy.

BACKSEAT

Also nates.

BACKSET

A relapse of a disease.

BAD MEDICINE

A Native American belief in the supernatural power of a person or thing to bring harm to others.

BALNEOTHERAPY

Also water cure. The treatment of disease by baths taken in the sea or in mineral springs.

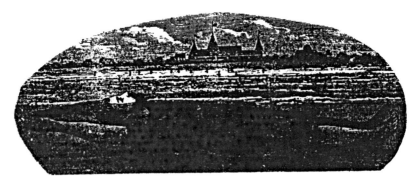

BALSAM OF MYRRH

A thick gummy juice from a tree native to Arabia. It was taken orally for pectoral affections and applied locally for ulcers, especially those found in the mouth and on the lips.

BANDY-LEGGED

Also bowlegged.

BARBER-SURGEONS

Healers of medieval Europe. They treated minor wounds and sores and performed procedures for physicians, such as bleeding or scarification. Barber-surgeons antedated physicians.

BARBER'S POLE

The symbol of the barber-surgeons' trade. The pole represents the arm. The red stripes depict the bleeding skin. The white stripes depict the tourniquet. The gilt knob on top of the pole depicts the bowl used to catch the blood. The bowl was used by the barber for shaving as well as blood catching.

BARREN

Also unfruitful. Describes a woman unable to conceive children.

BASTARD MEASLES

Also German measles.

BATH

A remedy to prevent or treat illness used since antiquity. A bath was a medium in which the body was wholly or partly immersed. Baths were given in water, air, sun, sand, mud, or electricity. These media varied according to temperature, the form

In which they were applied to the body, the addition of other remedies, and the part to be bathed. Baths became a highly favored form of treatment in the late 1800s and continued until the mid-1900s. A 1944 medical resource listed over 120 types of baths to be used for therapeutic purposes.

MEDICAL, SURGICAL AND VAPOR BATH INSTITUTE.

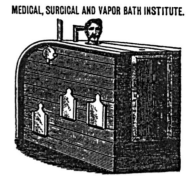

BATTLEY'S SEDATIVE DROPS
A patent remedy, consisting of a mixture of opium, water, and alcohol, used to reduce irritation or excitement.

BEARBERRY
Also mountain box. A low-lying, evergreen shrub native to Europe and Asia. Its leaves were believed to have astringent and tonic effects, and they were used mainly in the treatment of catarrhs of the urinary tract.

BEAR FAT
A greasy, semisolid substance extracted from bear meat and used by Native Americans for repelling insects and treating skin problems.

BEAR'S WEED
Also yerba santa.

BEECHAM'S PILLS
A patent remedy prepared according to a secret formula although it was known to contain aloes, ginger, and soap. It was acclaimed as a laxative.

BEESWAX
Also yellow wax.

BELLY-BOUND
Also costiveness.

BENZINE
A coal tar product that was inhaled for whooping cough, applied

to the skin for body lice, and taken orally for pork worm disease. It was prescribed by the "regulars" until the early 1900s.

BETHROOT
Also birthroot.

BEZOAR
A material formed into a solid mass found in the stomach and intestines of animals. It was believed to possess remedial value as an antidote to poisons and was used by the "regulars" until the early 1900s.

BIBULOUS
Having the ability to soak up liquid.
And inclined to tippling.

BILE
A thick, yellow-green fluid secreted by the liver and stored in the gall bladder where the color becomes greenish-brown.

BILIARY CONCRETIONS.
Also gall stones.

BILIOUS ATTACK
A digestive condition characterized by loss of appetite, constipation, headache, coated tongue, and malaise believed to be due to excessive secretion of bile.

BILIOUS FEVER
A remittent fever characterized by the vomiting of bile and, at times, accompanied by the yellowing of the skin.

BILIOUS TEMPERAMENT
Also choleric temperament.

BIRTHROOT
Also bethroot, Indian balm, trillium. An herbal remedy used by Native Americans and European Americans as an aid to childbirth.

BITTERS
A common name for a variety of medicinal drinks characterized

by a disagreeable taste and often containing alcohol. Used frequently as tonics, alteratives, or appetizers.

BITTER ASH
   Also quassia.

BITTERWOOD
   Also quassia.

BLACK BILE
   Also melancholer, melancholy. A dark colored "humoral" substance believed by ancient physicians to be from the spleen and stomach. See **GALEN** and **HIPPOCRATES**.

BLACK DEATH
   Also bubonic plague, oriental plague, the plague. An infectious disease carried by rats and transferred to man by the bite of the rat flea, it is characterized by high fever, swollen glands, and small bloody eruptions on the skin. It has been endemic in Asia. The first epidemic was noted in Europe in the 6th century and other epidemics have occurred since that time through the early part of the 20th century.

BLACK MAGIC
   Also sorcery.

BLACK PITCH
   Also coal tar.

BLEEDING BOWLS
   Containers made of tin-glazed earthen ware, pewter, or silver used to catch blood during the blood-letting process. Many had graduation lines marked on the inside to measure the amount of blood removed.

BLISTER BUG
   Also cantharides.

BLISTER FLY
   Also cantharides.

BLISTERING

The practice of applying irritants to the body. It was believed that internal diseases could be brought from deeper, diseased organs to the surface of the body and dispelled. Blistering was practiced from the Middle Ages through the 20th century.

BLISTERING CERATE [CERATA, CERATUM]

Also blistering plaster, cantharides plaster. A plaster consisting of dried cantharides spread in a base of fat or wax and applied to the skin. It was used to produce blisters in the treatment of deep-seated inflammations.

BLISTERING PLASTER

Also blistering cerate.

BLOOD

The vital fluid that circulates through the heart, arteries, and veins.

And a "humoral" substance believed by ancient physicians to come from the brain. See **GALEN** and **HIPPOCRATES**.

BLOODLETTING

The removal of blood from body as a therapeutic measure. Small amounts were removed by cupping, leeching, or scarification. Larger amounts were removed by directly opening a vein. A treatment dating back to the 4th century B.C. In the 18th century it was believed by some "regulars" that erratic motion of blood in the body was the cause of disease. If the pulse of the patient was felt to be "full and tense" then he was bled. It was considered necessary to relieve this tension or "boiling blood" for any cure to be effective.

BLOOD POISONING

Also pyemia.

BLOODSUCKER

Also leech.

BLOODY FLUX

Also dysentery.

BLOWING

An indirect reference used by European Americans to describe a

Native American belief in one form of the "bad medicine" of European Americans which brought illness and death. That is, European American visitors sent out double messages, "blowing hot and cold." Believed to be taken from the old fable of a visitor who mystified his host by blowing on his fingers to warm them and on his soup to cool it.

And a name for several methods of treatment used by the Cherokee medicine man. Most common was the method in which the medicine man took medicine into his mouth and then blew it over the body of the sick person. Other techniques included rubbing medicine on the sick person followed by the medicine man breathing on the person and blowing pipe tobacco smoke directly against an aching tooth.

BLUE LIGHT BATH
An electric light bath with blue light rays used to treat cases of neurosis by the "regulars" during the 19th and early 20th centuries.

BLUE-MASS
Also blue pill. A dose of mercury.

BLUE PILL
Also blue-mass.

BLUTREINIGUNGSMITTEL
Herbs used during spring rituals held by the Pennsylvania Germans to "thin their blood" and thus remain well. Some of those herbs were sassafras, sarsaparilla, and burdock. They were chosen for their red color and/or bitter taste, in the belief that these qualities indicated strong medicine.

BOAT-BELLY
The sunken appearance of the abdomen in emaciated individuals.

BOCO [BOKO]
Also houngan.

BODY BAKE
Also Turkish body bake. An application of very hot air achieved by enclosing the body in a lined, heated metal box. It was

used along with mercury in the treatment of syphilis by the "regulars" in the 19th and early 20th centuries.

BODY SNATCHERS
Also sack-'em-up-men.

BOIL
Also furuncle. A painful deep-seated skin eruption characterized by inflammation and a pustulous core.

BOILING
Also gallop. The bubbling action of a liquid when heated to a certain temperature.

BOILING BLOOD
An erratic condition of the blood characterized by increased motion and heat generated by blockages in the circulatory system. The heat caused inflammation of the surrounding area. A belief of the "regulars" in the 18th century; the treatment was blood-letting.

BOLD HIVES
Also croup.

BONDE-DOKTOR [DOKTER]
A Scandinavian word for doctors in the 19th century using herbal remedies and serving peasants.

BONESET
Also Indian sage, thoroughwort. A plant whose leaves and flowering tops were used as an herbal remedy. The Native Americans and colonial European Americans believed it to be a cure-all.

BOTANICAL MEDICINE
A system for the prevention and treatment of disease using remedies of plant origin only. It reached its greatest scope during the first half of the 19th century. The first healers were herb and root doctors. After 1845 many botanical medical colleges were opened but few remained viable. Botanical medicine melded with the "regulars" after the Civil War and "eclectic" medicine came into existence.

BOTTLE INHALER

A bottle half filled with a mixture of hot water and an expectorant. A person breathed the steam from the bottle as a treatment for croup.

BOTTLE NOSE

Also acne rosacea, brandy face, brandy nose, rosy drop, spider cancer, toper's nose, whiskey nose. A chronic disease marked by flushing of the skin on the nose, forehead, and cheeks and followed by red coloration due to dilation of the facial blood vessels accompanied by skin disturbances. Later the skin of the nose becomes thick and hard. It was believed to be caused by excessive intake of alcoholic beverages.

BOWLEGGED

Also bandy-legged. A condition in which the lower limbs curve outward.

BRACER

Also tonic.

BRAIDISM

Also animal magnetism.

And the hypnotic state produced by fixation of the eye on a shining object, as noted by Dr. James Braid in 1842.

BRAN

Outer shells of edible grains, e.g., wheat and rye.

BRANDY FACE

Also bottle nose.

BRANDY NOSE

Also bottle nose.

BRANKS

Also scolding bridle. A metal, bridle-like, medieval instrument placed on the heads of argumentative women to muzzle that behavior.

And, in medicine, mumps.

BRASH
Also water brash.

BRASS FOUNDER'S AGUE
Also metal-fume fever.

BRAUCHING
Also powwowing.

BRAUN
Also erythema diffusum. A condition characterized by a rash similar to that found in scarlatina except that it usually covered the entire body. It was frequently found in patients with influenza, typhus fever, typhoid fever, and other kinds of sepsis.

BREAKBONE FEVER
Also dengue.

BREAST
Also mamma.

BREATHING A VEIN
Bloodletting in the arm. A treatment used for the relief of apoplexy.

BRIGHT'S DISEASE
Also albuminuria, essential nephritis, kidney disease. A diffuse, progressive, degenerative disease of the kidney characterized by dropsy of the upper and lower parts of the body. It ranked high as a cause of death during the 18th, 19th, and early 20th centuries.

BRIMSTONE
Also sulfur. A yellowish, nonmetallic element with many applications, including being melted and cast in cylindrical molds for medicinal use.

BRONCHOCELE
Also struma.
And, in the mid-1900s, dilation of one of the smaller airway branches (bronchiole) into the lungs.

BROOM'S ANTIHYDROPIC TINCTURE
A patent remedy that claimed to be the cure for dropsy. It was produced in the South during the 1860s.

BRUJA (female), **BRUJO** (male)
Spanish American practitioners of sorcery.

BUBOES [BUBO, BUBOS]
Also St. Roch's disease. Inflammation and swelling of the lymph glands in the groin or armpit usually following venereal infection.

BUBONIC PLAGUE
Also black death.

BUCKTHORN
A common name for a group of small trees and shrubs of which some are native to California. Until the late 18th century the bark of two species was used to produce cascara sagrada. Then one species was found to have bark which was particularly effective as a cathartic and is now used to produce cascara sagrada. The other had bark that was found useful in the treatment of rheumatism.

BUFFALO BALL
A smooth, round mass resembling a ball, formed from body accretions which become hard when removed from the buffalo's stomach. Native Americans of the Kiowa tribe believed that it protected them from being killed. They regarded it as the "medicine of life," and wore "the medicine stone" as a charm attached to a warhorse. Some were as large as an apple, about three inches in diameter. Similar to bezoar.

BUGS
Also insects. A general term applied to a variety of "minute animals" in the 19th century especially those infesting homes, bodies, heads, and beds. They were believed to be the cause of many diseases.

BUNCOMBE
Also bunk, bunkum, humbug, puffery. Empty talk or hype to inflate the value of something, such as patent medicines.

BUNDLE
Also medicine bag.

BUNK [BUNKUM]
Also buncombe.

BURDOCK
An herb whose root was used in the treatment of gout, scurvy, syphilis, and skin diseases.

BURKING
The murder of an individual in such a way that it causes little destruction to the corpse, because the intent of the murderer is to sell the body to a medical school for dissection. It was named after William Burke who was punished for this crime in 1829.

BUTTOCKS
Also nates.

BUYING THE DISEASE
Also inoculation.

CACHET
Also capsule.

CAFFEINE [CAFFEA, CAFFEIN]
A substance found in the coffee bean, cola nut, and tea leaf. It acts as a stimulant, predominantly on the brain but also on the heart.

CALOMEL
Also mercurous chloride. A metallic remedy believed to be useful in the treatment of syphilis, gastro-intestinal problems and as an alterative. Evidence of the drug's effectiveness was noted by the excess production of saliva. A commonly prescribed remedy of the "regulars" in the 19th and early 20th centuries.

CALUMET
A highly decorated ceremonial pipe of the Native Americans used only on special religious and state occasions.

CAMISOLE
A straitjacket used for the restraint of violent persons. 19th century.

CAMOMILE
Also chamomile, little apple, manzanilla, mayweed. A term used to indicate two plants commonly known as Roman chamomile and German chamomile both believed to have gentle healing qualities. Spanish Americans in the southwest used the herb for colic and other infant ailments. German Americans believed that the herb could be used for all illnesses. In medieval England they were used as "strewing" herbs to freshen the air.

CAMP FEVER
Also typhus.

CAMPHOR
A gum obtained from an evergreen tree native to China and Japan. In the 19th century, it was used internally to treat hysteria, nervousness, and severe diarrhea. Poisoning was not uncommon. Externally, it was used as a counter-irritant for rheumatism and respiratory conditions. It is still in use today. Vick's VapoRub® contains 4.73% camphor and is labeled as a decongestant/cough suppressant.

CANCER
In the 18th century, a term that denoted external non-malignant sores.
And, in the 19th century, a tumor that destroys life.
And, in the 20th century, any malignant tumor.

CANTHARIDES [CANTHARIS]
Also blister bug, blister fly, Spanish fly. The dried body of a species of beetle. It was used externally as a counter-irritant and blistering agent and internally as a genitourinary irritant or aphrodisiac.

CANTHARIDES PLASTER
Also blistering cerate.

CAPSULE
A pharmaceutical name for a small gelatinous shell divided so that the parts fit together as a box and cover. It is used for the administration of disagreeable tasting medicines.

And also cachet. A pharmaceutical name for the container used to encapsulate a drug made by placing a drug between two layers of wafers or rice paper and then sealing the edges.

And also perloid. A proprietary name for a capsule.

CARBO
Also charcoal.

CARBOLIC ACID
Also phenol. A coal tar product used mainly for its powerful germicidal property. Externally, it was used to clean surgeries and rooms in which the sick were housed. Everything was cleaned, including bedding, clothing, and instruments. It was also used to burn away infected tissue in skin affections. Internally, it was used to treat typhoid fever, whooping cough, and dyspepsia.

CARBUNCLE
A firm, deep, painful suppurative inflammation of tissue under the skin. It differs from a boil in that it is larger and has multiple points of suppuration.

And, until the 19th century, the term used to denote the condition thereafter known as anthrax.

CARNATION
The natural color of flesh/skin for Caucasian European Americans.

CAROLINA PINK
Also pinkroot.

CASCARA SAGRADA
Also sacred bark. The bark of a California buckthorn shrub originally used by Native Americans as a remedy for constipation. It was marketed by an American drug company in 1877 and was believed to be the most widely used laxative in the world.

CATAMENIA
Also courses.

CATAPLASM
Also poultice. A soft pulp-like mass made by mixing bran or meal with water. Used for the application of heat, moisture and/or local stimulation to achieve comfort and/or cure in an affected part of the body.

CATARRH
Inflammation of a mucous membrane with discharge.
And the inflammation of the tubules of the kidney and the air-sacs of the lungs.
And a term used with great frequency for two millennia to denote illness in general.

CATHARTIC
A remedy that produces emptying of the bowels.

CAUDLE
Also cordial. An alcoholic remedy given to newborns that were in need of stimulation to survive.

CAUL
Fetal membranes that can cover the head of the newborn at time of birth. It was believed to be a sign of good luck.

CELERY SEED
Also apium.

CERATE
A remedy consisting of oil or lard, mixed with wax or resin, to which various medicines were added. The consistency was firmer than an ointment and spread on linen cloth or leather by means of a spatula before application to the body.

CHAMOMILE
Also camomile.

CHANCROID
A local, venereal ulceration characterized by suppuration and

swelling of glands in the groin. In the past it was confused with the ulcer found in the primary stage of syphilis.

CHANGE
In the 19th century, a common term used for either the beginning or the cessation of the menstrual function.

CHANGE OF LIFE
Menopause, as often attended by signs of body disturbances, e.g., nervousness, agitation, and irritability.

CHARCOAL
Also carbo. A coal product distilled from wood after it is burned. It was used as a disinfectant and deodorizer, in poultices for wounds, and to dress ulcers. It was taken orally for gastrointestinal irritation.

CHARLATAN
Also quack.
And any "regular" who advertised his name and credentials in newspapers or community announcements, even if the credentials were valid.

CHARM
A word, phrase, action, gesture or object believed to have some supernatural power.

CHARPIE
A picked or shredded lint of linen for dressing wounds.

CHEMIST SHOP
A British term for a pharmacy.

CHICKEN POX
Also varicella.

CHIGGER [CHIGOE]
Also jigger.

CHILBLAIN
Also pernio. A chronic condition characterized by inflammation

and swelling of the skin due to exposure to severe cold. The skin would itch and/or burn and was usually worse at night.

CHILDBED FEVER
Also puerperal fever.

CHILD-CROWING
Also laryngeal stridor. The harsh, high-pitched sounds of children with a breathing difficulty. A sudden upper airway spasm made it difficult to breath and caused this sound on inhalation. It was often found in children that had rickets.

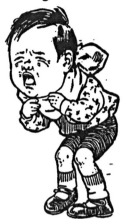

CHILD-NURSE
Also nursemaid. Usually a young woman employed in some homes to tend children in the 18th and 19th centuries. The term was replaced by "nanny" and "governess" in the mid-1900s.

CHIN SANG
Also ginseng.

CHINESE CUPPING
An ancient treatment for disease in which the tip of a horn was cut off to open the horn completely. The wide end was applied to the skin, and air was sucked out of the horn, which was then plugged with a finger to maintain suction.

CHINESE IRONING TREATMENT
Also ironing treatment. A remedy for local pain that consisted of placing herbs on the part of the body to be treated then covering them with a cloth that was heated by an iron or hot-water container.

CHINESE MEDICINE MEN
They were ancient healers or shamans whose practice, according to the "oracle bones," included the healing of injuries and skin diseases. They used magic in their healing efforts, and created stone needles for opening boils.

CHINESE MOON THERAPY

Also moon therapy. A remedy, consistent with passive Yin, for women. They were exposed to the moon's energy which they collected through yellow paper on which magic signs were inscribed.

CHINESE REMEDIAL MASSAGE

Also remedial massage. A remedy based on the belief that man's original medical tool is the hand that reflexively responds to pain on any part of the body to protect or rub. They believe that pressing and rubbing tones the body and thrusting and rolling sedates the body. Massage of certain parts of the body relieves specific problems. For example, massage of the umbilical area is used for abdominal pain.

CHINESE SUN THERAPY

Also sun therapy. A remedy, consistent with active Yang, for men. They were exposed to the sun's energy which they collected through a red or green paper containing a magic formula.

CHIROMANCY

Also palmistry. The practice of the reading of the palm to predict future health and wealth.

CHIROPRACTIC

A system of therapy founded in 1895 by a grocer named Daniel David Palmer. He believed that a flow of energy from the brain was necessary to maintain health and that interference with this flow produced disease. The spine was considered the area responsible for interfering with the flow. The treatment was spinal manipulation. The part of the spine in need of adjustment was palpated by the therapist and moved into correct alignment to allow for energy flow. In the early to mid-1900s, "nerve impulses" replaced "flow of energy" in chiropractic doctrine. The spine, joints, and muscle tissue are manipulated to return function of the nerves. Manipulation is supplemented with physical therapy, exercise, and dietary recommendations.

CHIRURGERY

Also surgery.

CHIRURGION [CHIRURGEON]

Also surgeon.

CHIRYO
A Japanese American remedy which consisted of the application of dried and burning moss to the body.

CHLOROSIS
Also green sickness. An anemia that affected girls at the age of puberty. Characterized by a greenish color of the skin, gastric problems, and menstrual disturbances.

CHOLER
Also yellow bile.

CHOLERA
Also Asiatic cholera, scourge of nations, white flux. An acute infectious disease characterized by severe diarrhea, vomiting, and inflammation of the colon. Initially noted in India, the disease is of great antiquity. The first great epidemic occurred throughout Asia and Africa in 1817 and reached North America in 1832. It remains endemic in Asia and sporadic epidemics occur throughout the world.

CHOLERA INFANTUM
Also cholera morbus, infantile diarrhea, summer complaint. A disease of infants and young children characterized by vomiting, severe diarrhea, and fever. It was of short duration and death frequently occurred within three to five days. It was common among the poor and hand fed infants, and was found frequently in summer and early autumn.

CHOLERA MORBUS
Also cholera infantum.

CHOLERA POWDER
A remedy for the prevention and treatment of cholera consisting of calomel, pepper, and camphor prescribed by the "regulars" during the 19th and early 20th centuries.

CHOLERA PREVENTION BOX
A large wooden closet in which an individual stood, body encased and head outside, while air-bathing in fumes of lime and carbolic acid. It was believed that this treatment would protect the

traveler from cholera in the area being visited. A post-Civil War device.

CHOLERIC TEMPERAMENT

Also bilious temperament. A name for the disposition of one who is quick to anger. Some believed hair growing low on the forehead was a sign of this humor, which predominated over the other temperaments: melancholic, phlegmatic, and sanguine. See **GALEN**.

CHOREA

Also St. Vitus' dance.

CHRISTIAN SCIENCE

Also "Church of Christ, Scientist," Eddyism. A religion and system of healing founded by Mary Baker Eddy in 1866. Based on her interpretation of the Bible, the cause of disease and sin was mental rather than physical and could be eliminated by spiritual treatment without medical help. The "divine science" of "mind-healing" comes from the "divine Mind." A metaphysical concept, mind-healing consisted of helping the sick person into the spiritual mindset needed to heal oneself. A common way to acquire this mindset was through the study of *Science and Health*, a textbook written by the founder.

CHRONIC DERMATITIS

Also eczema.

CHRONIC DISEASE

An illness characterized by slow progress and long duration.

CHURCH OF CHRIST, SCIENTIST

Also Christian Science.

CHYRURGERY

Also surgery.

CHYRURGION [CHYRURGEON]

Also surgeon.

CINCHONA BARK

Also Jesuits' bark.

CINNAMON WOOD
Also sassafras tree.

CIVIL WAR (THE)
The war between the States from April 1861 to April 1865.

CLAP
Also gonorrhea.

CLARY
A remedial drink consisting of a clear mixture of spices, wine, and honey.

CLERGYMAN'S SORE THROAT
An impairment of the voice due to excessive or improper use of the voice. Can also be caused by excessive use of tobacco or liquor.

CLIMACTERIC INSANITY
Also melancholia. Mental illness brought on by the change of life (menopause).

CLOTTERING [CLOTTING]
Also coagulation, curdling. The formation of soft solids out of semi-thick fluids, such as milk or blood.

CLOVE
The tree of tropical countries whose dried unopened flower buds were used as a home remedy for toothaches.
And the spice consisting of the dried unopened flower buds of the clove tree. A bruised clove would be held in the mouth to extract its anesthetic effect. It was prescribed for digestive problems and as an aromatic stimulant by the "regulars" until the mid-1900s.

CLOWNISM
A display of gestures and facial contortions that were seen in some forms of hysteria.

CLYSMA
Also clyster.

CLYSTER
Also enema, clysma, glister. A liquid injection into the rectum as

a purgative or as a medicine. A form of treatment known since antiquity.

COAGULATION
Also clottering.

COAL FOODS
Foods that form the main meal of any regular meal, such as meat, bread, rice, and cheese. Early 1900s.

COAL GAS
A vapor produced by the distillation of coal used for illumination, cooking, and heating.

COAL OIL
Also kerosene.

COAL TAR
Also black pitch. A thick, black liquid formed as a by-product in the distillation of coal gas. Used in many dyes, natural remedies, and synthetic remedies.

COCA
The leaves of a shrub that grew wild in South America. Native Americans chewed the leaves to ward off hunger when working without food. Believed to have been regarded as a divine plant by the Incas and used in their religious ceremonies. The "regulars" considered it to be useful as a tonic and cerebral stimulant until the mid-1900s.

COCAINE [COCAINA]
The active element found in coca. It has been used as a stimulant, narcotic, and local anesthetic by the "regulars." Habitual use of cocaine was called cocainism.

COCAINISM
The prolonged, habitual use of cocaine that was characterized by insomnia and emaciation.

COCKLEBUR
Also stitchwort.

COD
Also scrotum.

CODSWALLOP
Also quack.

COFFEE
Also Kaffee. The dried seed of a shrub native to Africa and known since the 6th century. The seed is roasted and ground and used in an infusion to produce the drink called "coffee." Coffee contains the stimulant caffeine. Medicinally, it was used to treat coughing attacks, headaches, and opium poisoning; it was also used as a disinfectant and deodorizing material. In the 19th and early 20th centuries, it was considered, along with tea, by some physicians and religious groups to be a habit-forming drug in the same category as alcohol and tobacco.

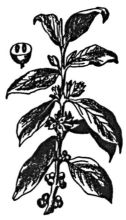

— Branch of a coffee plant with bunches of coffee berries near the bottom.

COLA NUT
Also kola nut.

COLD AIR BATH
A treatment for prevention and cure of disease. It consisted of a hard body rub with toweling and exposure to the air for half a minute in cold weather and three to four minutes in warm weather.

COLD BATH
A treatment that was believed to be a powerful stimulant to the nervous system as well as a fever reducing remedy. The water was kept between 32° and 70° Fahrenheit.

COLD TOWEL RUB
Also towel bath.

COLIC
A severe gripping pain in the intestines caused by spasms of the intestinal wall.

And any severe sudden muscular contraction of the abdomen.

COLLYRIUM
An eyewash or an eye lotion.

COLONIAL TIMES
Generally, the period of time during which the original colonies were settled until after the Revolutionary War: approximately, 1600 through the late 1700s.

COMA VIGIL
Also morbid vigilance.

COMFIT
A dry sweetmeat, especially one consisting of a piece of fruit or a medicinal solid coated with sugar.

COMMON HOUSE FLY
A two winged insect, discovered in the 19th century to be a mechanical carrier of diseases, e.g., typhoid, cholera, dysentery, and the plague.

CONDOMS
Also French letters.

CONFECTION
A medicinal preparation in which the drug is mixed with honey or syrup as a preservative or in order to provide an easier means of administrating.

CONFECTIONER'S DISEASE
A disease affecting confectionery workers in which their finger nails fell off.

CONGELATION
Also freezing, frostbite. The process of hardening due to exposure of parts of the body to the cold.

And coagulation.

CONJURE
Also powwow. The act of summoning supernatural help or healing in the belief that supernatural forces could be mediated through objects and human beings. The term was used most often in the South and by African Americans.

CONJURER
Also medicine man.
And one who summons supernatural help.

CONSTIPATION
Also costiveness.

CONSTITUTIONAL PATHOLOGY
A general term used to indicate predisposition to illness.

CONSUMPTION
Also phthisis.

CONSUMPTIVE'S WEED
Also yerba santa.

CONTAGIOUS
Communicable or transmissible by direct or indirect contact.

CONTAGIOUS DISEASE
An illness that is communicated by contact with an individual suffering from it, or contact with bodily secretions from that individual, or contact with an object used by the individual. Diptheria and smallpox are examples. Most diseases are infectious, though not necessarily contagious. Others, e.g. scabies, are contagious but not infectious.

CONTAGIOUS MAGIC
Also folk magic.

CONTINUED FEVER
Also variola.

CORDIAL
Also caudle.

CORN SILK
Also zea. The green hair-like pistils of the corn plant. A Native American remedy used by the "regulars" in the treatment of urinary conditions and cardiac dropsy.

CORN SMUT
A fungus found on corn. Used for stimulating contractions in childbirth and to control hemorrhage.

CORROBORANT
A remedy that has strong tonic action.

COSTIVENESS
Also belly-bound, constipation. A condition in which the bowels are evacuated at long intervals or with difficulty.

COTTON
A plant whose white, fluffy, fibrous covering of its seed has been used extensively for fabrics. In colonial times it was chewed for toothaches and decoctions of the powdered root were used as a stimulant and an emmenagogue.

COUNTERIRRITANT
An agent that causes superficial irritation of the skin used to relieve an inflammation of deeper structures. It was believed that it would substitute the lesser pain of the irritant for the greater pain in the body.

COURSES
Also catamenia, menses, sick, the curse, unwell. The monthly discharge of bloody fluid from the genital canal of women.

COW COLD
Also autumnal catarrh.

CRAB'S CLAWS
A remedy made up of finely powdered crab's claws used to relieve acid stomach.

CRAB'S EYE
Also eye stone.

CRAZINESS
Also madness.

CROUP
Also bold hives, hives, trachitis. A disease of the larynx and trachea in the upper airways of children. Characterized by a harsh, ringing cough and difficulty in breathing.

CROUP KETTLE
A vessel with a long spout and an attached rubber hose by which steam was sent to the patient. Often the patient was inside a tent erected over a bed. The water in the vessel contained a small piece of lime. Used to treat croup and diphtheria.

CROWD POISON
An unstable organic matter in the air of poorly ventilated places where many persons were congregated.

CROWE'S BEAK
A forceps for sewing wounds in the 16th century.

CROWE'S BILL
An instrument for removing stones from the body in the 16th century.

CUPPING
A treatment to raise a blister or promote bleeding which involved the application to the skin of a small container from which the air had been removed either by heating or with a special suction device. Except in dry cupping, this treatment often involved incision or scarification as well. Prior to the advent of the cupping glass, suction was achieved by sucking the air out through an animal horn or by using the mouth alone. See **CHINESE CUPPING**.

CUPPING GLASS
The small bell-shaped glass applied to the skin after a vacuum was created. Used in the treatment known as cupping.

CUPPING GLASS

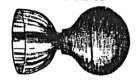

CURANDERAS (female), **CURANDEROS** (male)
Spanish American or Mexican American healers.

CURDLING
Also clottering.

CURE
A system of treatment.
And the successful treatment of a disease.

CURSE (THE)
Also courses.

CURSE OF EVE
Labor pains during childbirth.

CUTTING OF THE TEETH
Also teething.

DANDY FEVER
Also dengue.

DAYMARE
A condition similar to a nightmare but occurring while the individual was awake.

DEACONESSES
Nurses that were trained under the auspices of the Protestant church in Germany. They were the first nurses to receive formal training to care for the sick--a three year program. The first student was admitted in 1836. They came to America in 1849 and opened a hospital in Pennsylvania.

DEAD AGUE
Also dumb ague.

DEAD-BORN
Also stillborn.

DEAD PALSY
A loss of motion and feeling in a part of the body.

DEATH STRUGGLE
Also agony.

DECOCTION
A liquid preparation, believed to contain the essential medicinal elements of a plant, obtained by boiling the plant substances in water.

DECUMBITURE
The act of taking to one's bed when ill.

DEFICIENCY DISEASE
A generic term for diseases caused by a lack of an essential element in the diet.

DEMENTIA
A form of insanity characterized by irreversible deterioration of intellectual faculties, reasoning skills, and memory.

DENGUE
Also breakbone fever, dandy fever, scarlatina rheumatica. An acute infectious disease characterized by fever, severe pain in bones, joints, muscles and, at times, a skin eruption. It is found in tropical and subtropical climates.

DENTISTRY
The care of teeth in colonial times consisted of the removal of bad teeth and the making of artificial teeth. The country doctor and itinerant merchant provided dental care as a sideline to their usual trade.

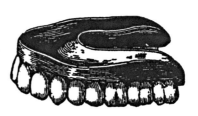

The first dental college was opened in 1839 and dentistry as a separate specialty of the "regulars" became an accepted form of care in the late 1800s.

DEW ITCH
Also ground itch.

DIARRHEA
A bowel condition characterized by increased frequency and lessened consistency of fecal discharge.

DIPHTHERIA
Also membranous angina. An acute infectious disease characterized by inflammation and the formation of a thick covering on the mucous membranes of the throat and nose. General symptoms included fever, weakness of the heart, and rapidly developing anemia, later understood to be caused by poisons given off from the bacteria responsible for the initiation of the disease. Severe epidemics were reported in different parts of Europe during the 16th, 17th, and 18th centuries. It was a disease of childhood and very fatal. Outbreaks continued throughout the world until the middle of the 20th century.

DIPHTHERITIC CROUP
Also laryngeal diphtheria, membranous croup. An acute, contagious disease preceded by diphtheria of the throat and/or nose and characterized by severe breathing problems due to the thick, obstructive covering on the membranes of the throat and/or nose.

DIRT EATING
Also geophagism, mal d'estomac. The act of eating dirt or clay. It was found in advanced cases of hookworm disease.

DISCUSS'
To cause a tumor or other lesion to disappear.

DISCUTIENT
A remedy that causes unhealthy matter formed in a diseased state to disappear. Poulticing and fomentation are examples of discutients.

DISEASE CAUSES: NATIVE AMERICAN
Native Americans believed that illness was caused by the presence of a material object in the body of the sick person or as an effect of the absence of the soul from the body of the sick person. Sorcerers caused these conditions, and medicine men were responsible for treating these conditions by seeking the help of superhuman powers.

DISEASE OF HISPANIOLA
Also syphilis.

DISTEMPER
A generic term used until the 20th century to indicate a diseased state in man. Since then, it has been used to indicate an infectious disease found in animals.

DIVINE RETRIBUTION
An ancient belief, well established in the Old Testament, that sickness was a punishment sent by God for breaking a religious law. It is believed by some biblical historians that adherence to this belief delayed the Jewish people from seeking out natural causes of disease.

DIVINES
A name given to religious groups which incorporated healing powers in their religious practice, such as the Society of Friends, also known as Quakers, and Methodists.

DOCHMIASIS [DOCHMIOSIS]
Also hookworm disease.

DOCTOR'S SUCKING GLASS
Also glass leech.

DOCTRINE OF SIGNATURES
The theory that medicinal uses of plants and other objects can be determined from their appearance. For example, the yellow color of saffron indicated its use for jaundice, and the spotted skin of the lizard indicated its use for tumors.

DOG DAYS
The period in the year between early July and early September.

DOG HUNGER
A continuous craving for food.

DOMESTIC MEDICINE
Also self-dosage. The home treatment of illnesses without the advice of a physician.

DOTAGE
In the 16th century, a form of madness that was mild, continuous, and without fever or ague.

And, in the 18th century, a harmless senility found in the aged.

DOUBLING OF THE JOINTS
Also rickets.

DOVER'S POWDER
A popular remedy prescribed by the "regulars" used for the relief of the aches and pain of fever patients. It was a mixture of opium, ipecac, and milk sugar. The opium sedated, the ipecac reduced fever through sweating, and the milk sugar sweetened the taste.

DRACHM [DRAM]
A measurement--the eighth part of an ounce.

DRAPET
An obsolete term for cloth or covering.

DRAPETOMANIA
In the early 1800s a term to describe a disorder first noted among slaves because it caused them to run away. Literally, fear of being covered with cloth.

And, in the late 1800s, a form of madness characterized by a morbid desire to wander from home.

DRASTIC
A powerful and irritating cathartic causing a watery fecal discharge.

DREAM FULFILLMENT
Also Indian dream fulfillment. Native Americans believed that desires revealed in dreams had to be satisfied in order to cure an illness.

DRIED STOMACH
The dried, powdered and defatted wall of the stomach of the hog. Used in the treatment of anemia, particularly pernicious anemia.

DRIVEL
Also slaver.

DROPPING
A euphemistic term for infant death due to abandonment in the 18th and 19th centuries.

DROPSY
Also edema, hydrops, hydropsy. A condition characterized by swelling due to watery accumulation in any of the tissues or cavities of the body.

DROPSY OF THE CHEST
Also hydrothorax.

DRUGGIST
In colonial times a druggist was a person who imported drugs and sold them wholesale. In the 1800s the druggist became known as an apothecary or pharmacist who prepared remedies on prescription of a physician and, oftentimes, prescribed and sold remedies retail.

DRUMMER
Also hawker, puffer. A seller of patent medicines along with other items that were not generally available to communities.

DRY BELLYACHE
A condition, usually due to the use of lead given for treatment of a disease, such as worm infestation, and characterized by severe abdominal pain with constipation.

DRY CUPPING
A form of counterirritation in which the blood was drawn to the surface by means of a cup. The skin was not incised.

DUCK'S FOOT
Also May apple.

DUFFY'S ELIXIR

A patent remedy for all infant ills. It was made up of senna, jalap, aniseed, caraway seeds and juniper berries which were steeped in alcohol and then mixed with molasses and water. Mid-18th century.

DUMB AGUE

Also dead ague, irregular ague, latent ague, masked ague. A form of malaria characterized by irregular attacks of fever without chills.

DYSENTERY

Also bloody flux. An inflammatory disease of the large intestine believed to be infectious and characterized by pain and the frequent passage of small amounts of stool mixed with blood and mucus. It was known by both Hippocrates and Galen. The term was used generally until the 1870s when the specific varieties, amebic and bacillary, were identified.

DYSPEPSIA

Also the plague of civilization.

DYSURY [DYSURIA]

Painful or difficult urination.

EARTH BANDAGE

A treatment in which moist earth or clay was placed directly in or on a wound and then tied in place with a linen bandage.

EARTH CLOSET

Also privy.

EARTH COMPRESS

A remedy in which earth or clay was applied cold over an affected area, covered with a layer of cotton or wool, and bandaged to hold it in place.

ECLAMPSIA
An acute nervous affection characterized by convulsions and loss of consciousness.

ECLAMPSIA PUERPERALIS
A convulsion that occurs in the mother late in pregnancy, during labor, or shortly after delivery. It was believed to be caused by kidney malfunction.

ECLECTIC MEDICINE
A method of medical practice taught in some medical schools in America after the Civil War. The keystone of the method was botanical medicine. Symptoms were to be principally treated using specific plant remedies for known specific diseases. An important outcome of this approach was the introduction of standardization of drug dosage, i.e., specification of the amount of drug to be given for each specific disease.

ECLECTIC PRACTITIONERS
Physicians in America that believed in specific definitive remedies and the use of preparations made from indigenous plants.
And physicians that freed themselves from the existing sects and selected the perceived best from each.

ECLEGM
Also electuary.

ECZEMA
Also chronic dermatitis, vesicular dermatitis. An inflammation of the skin characterized by lesions that vary in appearance from red, slightly swollen, and moist to small watery blisters to small pus-containing blisters. Itching is intense, and it can appear on any part of the body. The cause is unknown. In the 19th century, it was believed to be caused by eating pork, Bright's disease, gout, and/or heat. Certain occupations, such as mason, laundress, and baker, were believed to be more prone to contracting eczema. Treatment included cleansing with tar soap, hot sponging, prolonged cold applications, and ointments containing sulfur. It was classified as chronic dermatitis in the mid-1900s.

EDEMA
Also dropsy.

EDDYISM
Also Christian Science.

EGYPTIAN CHLOROSIS
Also hookworm disease.

ELECTRIC BATH
A treatment in which the patient was placed on an insulated stool and charged with positive or negative electricity. It was used for treatment of neuralgias and menstrual problems.

ELECTROPHOTOTHERAPY
A treatment, usually for skin conditions, using an electric light.

ELECTROTHERAPY [ELECTROTHERAPEUTICS]
The use of electricity in the treatment of disease. Electric impulses were directed to various parts of the body to stimulate muscular reactions.

ELECTUARY
Also eclegm. A soft mass containing powdered medicine mixed with sugar, honey, and water.

ELL
An English measurement equal to 1 1/4 yards.
And a French measurement equal to 1 1/2 yards.

EMETIC
Also vomitory.

EMMENAGOGUE
A remedy that stimulates menstrual flow.

EMPIRIC
Also quack.
And a healer who learned the trade through an apprenticeship with botanical practitioners or simply through experience. The "regulars" considered empirics to be quacks.

EMPLASTRUM
Also plaster.

ENCEPHALOMALACIA
Also softening of the brain. A progressive form of insanity characterized by general paralysis and loss of reason and memory.

ENDEMIC
Describes the prevalence of a disease when it is found in a certain place more or less continuously.

ENEMA
Also clyster.
And also Indian enema. Native American tubes and bulb syringes for rectal purgation were made of bladders of animals and hollow leg bones of birds or of hollow rushes. They created this equipment and used it to treat diarrhea, constipation, and hemorrhoids (piles).

ENGLISH DISEASE
Also syphilis.

ENGLISH SWEAT
Also sweating disease.

ENGRAFTING [IN GRAFTING]
Also inoculation.

ENLIGHTENMENT (THE)
An 18th century philosophical movement in Europe that called into question the supernatural aspects of folk medicine and gave rise to the application of terms such as "superstition" and "quackery" to all forms of folk medicine.

ENTERIC FEVER
Also typhoid fever.

ENTERITIS
An inflammation of the intestine--mainly the small intestine. A condition that has been attributed to many causes, including teething, a sudden drop in temperature, poor environment and neurosis.

EPHEMERA
An illness that lasts less than 24 hours.

EPHEMERAL FEVER
Also feveret.

EPIDEMIC
Prevalence of a disease that affects many people and/or is spread over a wide area.

EPIDEMIC CATARRH
Also influenza.

EPIDEMIC ROSEOLA
Also German measles.

EPIDERMIS
Also scarfskin.

EPILEPSY
Also falling sickness, the sacred disease. A chronic nervous disorder characterized by attacks of unconsciousness and/or convulsions. It was often associated in the later stages with mental disturbance. It has been known since antiquity.

EPILEPSY OF THE LUNG
Also asthma.

EQUINIA
Also glanders.

ERGOT
A fungus that grows on grain, especially rye. Prior to the 19th century, it was believed to be the seed of a grain altered by an insect or an excess of heat and moisture. It causes contraction of the muscular coat of the small blood vessels carrying blood from the heart to the body. It was often used to control uterine bleeding after childbirth by midwives and the "regulars." It was also considered medically useful for reducing excessive amounts of blood in parts of the body, particularly the spine and the brain, until the mid-1900s. Migraines are currently treated with this drug.

ERGOTISM
Also St. Anthony's fire. A condition characterized by inflam-

mation and/or gangrenous skin conditions. In the 19th century it was found to be caused by eating bread made with grain containing the ergot fungus or by taking an overdose of the drug ergot.

ERUPTIVE DISEASES
A generic name covering chicken pox, measles, scarlet fever, and small pox.

ERYSIPELAS
Also St. Anthony's fire. A condition characterized by inflammation of the skin and subcutaneous tissues. The facial type followed a head cold. Redness started at the bridge of the nose and spread in a butterfly fashion over the cheeks. In the 19th century it was found to be an infectious disease.

ERYTHEMA DIFFUSUM
Also braun.

ESSENCE PEDDLER
A seller of peppermint and wintergreen extracts, and bitters in the 18th century. The bitters were in great demand in the countryside where they were mixed with the local homemade liquor as a tonic.

ESSENTIAL NEPHRITIS
Also Bright's disease.

ESTIVOAUTUMNAL FEVER
Also malaria.

EUROPEAN MANDRAKE
Also Satan's apple.

EVIL EYE
An ancient belief, found in many parts of the world, in the power of the human eye. Greek Americans believe that some people have the power to injure another merely by looking at them. This power may or may not be evident, either to observers or to the individual with the power.

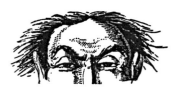

The evidence that the power has been used is noted by the harm done to another. A particularly unusual concern of those who believe in evil eye is that a child may be harmed by individuals with this power simply through the kindly remarks that this individual makes while looking at the child.

EXCREMENT
Also feces.

EYEBALL
Also apple of the eye.

EYE STONE
Also crab's eye. A small smooth shell or similar object used for removing foreign bodies from the eye.

FAINT
Also swoon.

FAITH HEALING
A method of curing sickness by prayer and/or religious rite.

FALLING OF THE FUNDAMENT
Also anal prolapse. The protrusion of the lower portion of the bowel through the anus.

FALLING SICKNESS
Also epilepsy.

FAMINE
A wide-spread scarcity of food. They were a frequent occurrence in the Mississippi Valley during the first half of the 1800s, and many African Americans died of starvation.

FAMINE FEVER
Also relapsing fever. An acute, infectious disease characterized

by fever, sweating, delirium, and spleen enlargement. The first attack lasted 5 to 6 days recurring after variable intervals two or more times. Conditions of over-crowding and lack of adequate food supply were believed to be the causative factors in the 19th century. In the early 20th century the bedbug and the louse were found to carry the disease.

FAN BATH
A treatment to reduce fever that involved promoting evaporation from a sheet covering the patient. The sheet was sprinkled with cold water and then used to provide gentle massage to the patient's extremities.

FARADIZATION
A form of electrotherapy. The use of an interrupted current for the stimulation of muscles and nerves. A patient would sit with his feet on a large electrode and another electrode would be applied to various parts of the body to be treated. Used in the 19th and early 20th centuries.

FARCY
Also glanders.

FEBRIFUGE
A remedy that reduces fever.

FEBRILE EXCITEMENT
The state of restlessness and irritability that sometimes accompanied a fever.

FEBRIS
Also fever.

FECES
Also excrement, ordure, siege. Normal bowel discharge.

FETISH
An image or object believed to be possessed of supernatural power and worshiped.

FETOR
An offensive odor.

FEVER

Also febris, pyrexia. A condition noted by great bodily heat and excessive thirst.

And, in the early 19th century, believed to be a disease state characterized by increased body heat, rapid pulse, loss of appetite, headache, and general malaise.

And, beginning in the late 19th century with the advent of thermometers adapted for medical use, a body temperature above the normal of 98.6º Fahrenheit.

FEVER AND AGUE

Also malaria.

FEVERET

Also ephemeral fever. A low fever lasting one or two days.

FEVERFEW

Also mutterkraut. A plant native to Europe. The whole plant, excluding the root, was used to make a bitter tonic for treating illnesses.

FEVER THERAPY

Also pyretotherapy. The treatment of disease by intermittent elevation of body temperature through electrical means or by inoculation of malarial organisms.

FILTH DISEASE

Also typhoid fever.

FIRING

A treatment for neuralgia and spinal irritation in which an iron disk that had been heated with boiling water was rapidly passed over the skin to cause blistering.

FIT [FITT]

An attack of an acute disease, or the sudden appearance of some sign, such as, a convulsion or epileptic seizure.

FLEA

Also jigger.

FLEAM
Also schnapper. A spring operated lancet.

FLEET MILK
Also skim milk.

FLOODING
Hemorrhage from the uterus.

FLUX
Also scouring.

FLYING BLISTER
A therapeutic blistering treatment of the skin that produced redness but not an actual blister.

FOLK HEALERS
Those individuals who practiced the art of curing disease without formal medical education. They worked in concert with their communities' ideas of life, death, health and illness.

FOLK MAGIC
Also contagious magic. A ritual in which the goal is to transfer an illness, directly or indirectly, to another person, animal, plant or object.

FOLK MEDICINE
A practice of health care outside the main stream of medicine using magic, herbs, roots, non-prescription drugs and folk healers to prevent illness and achieve and maintain health. The magical component was the essential part of the treatment plan.

FOMENTATION
Also poulticing. The application of heat, moisture and/or medicine to an affected part of the body to reduce pain and inflammation.

FOWLER'S SOLUTION
Also potassium arsenite solution. An arsenical used as a remedy for multiple disorders, including stomach disease, skin disease and fevers, in the 18th, 19th, and early 20th centuries. Arsenical

poisoning was a frequent, serious consequence of treatment with this remedy.

FRAMBESIA
Also yaws.

FREEZING
Also congelation.

FRENCH LETTERS
Also condoms. A prophylactic aid to sexual intercourse. A device made of sheep's intestine that was invented by Dr. Condom in London in the mid-1600s.

FRENCH MEASLES
Also German measles.

FRENZY
Also phrenzy.

FRET
To wear away by abrasive rubbing.

FRIGOTHERAPY
The treatment of disease by cold. Cold was used in various forms, such as baths, compresses, irrigations, lotions, and injections.

FROG-BELLY
The flaccid abdomen seen in children that had rickets.

FROSTBITE
Also congelation.

FULLER'S EARTH
A refined clay used as a dusting powder or applied with moisture as a poultice for skin conditions.

FUNGUS
A botanical group of plants without chlorophyll, varying greatly in size and form. It includes mushrooms, toadstools, molds, and a

large number of microscopic plants that grow upon other plants and animals. See **ERGOT** and **RINGWORM**.

FUR
A whitish coating of the tongue seen in indigestion and fevers.

FURFUR [FURFAIRE]
Any scaling of the skin, such as dandruff.

FURUNCLE
Also boil.

GAGROOT
Also pukeweed.

GALEN
A Greek physician born in 130 A.D. His written works on the use of herbs and roots in the practice of medicine was applied by other physicians until the Middle Ages. He is believed to have expanded the Hippocratic humoral theory with the idea that the four humors not only determine the health but also the temperament of the individual. The humors of Galen flowed from the corresponding "cardinal humors" of Hippocrates: blood/sanguine; black bile/melancholic; phlegm/phlegmatic; and yellow bile/choleric. See also **HIPPOCRATES** and **HUMOR**.

GALENE
Also theriaca.

GALLA [GALL]
Also gall, nutgall, oak apple. Abnormal oak tree growths due to the egg-laying of gallflies. Used to treat diarrhea and as a dye.

GALLOP
Also boiling.

GALLSTONES
Also biliary concretions. Hardened masses of mineral matter formed in the gall bladder and bile ducts.

GALVANISM
A form of electrotherapy. The use of direct current or electric current arising from chemical action to diagnose or cure disease. The current was passed through the body of the patient after it had been made to pass through the body of an attendant. Created in the latter half of the 18th century by Luigi Galvani.

GANGLION
Also weeping sinew.

GANGRENE
Also sphacelus.

GANGRENOUS EMPHYSEMA
Also malignant edema.

GANGRENOUS PHARYNGITIS
Also putrid sore throat.

GAOL FEVER
Also typhus.

GARROTE TOURNIQUET
Also Spanish windlass.

GAS GANGRENE
Also malignant edema.

GASTRIC JUICE
The secretions of the glands of the stomach. The gastric juices of animals were used for local application in cancers and gangrenous ulcers.

GATHERING
Inflamed breasts after childbirth.
And swelling due to pus lying under skin.

GENERAL ANEMIA
See **ANEMIA.**

GENERAL PARESIS
Also paretic dementia.

GEOPHAGISM
Also dirt eating.

GEORGET'S STUPIDITY
A mental condition that was characterized by simple confusion without hallucinations or delusions. A 19th century medical diagnosis.

GEREYTOUTE TEA
An African American traditional remedy for all illnesses. It was made of dried swimming bladders of fish, diluted juice of plants, wine, asafetida, and ground bone.

GERMAN DISEASE
Also syphilis.

GERMAN MEASLES
Also bastard measles, epidemic roseola, French measles, roetheln, rubella, rubeola. An acute, infectious, eruptive, disease characterized by its resemblance to both measles and scarlet fever, which are more severe. The symptoms include the catarrhal symptoms found in measles and the sore throat found in scarlet fever.

GERMICIDE
Also antiseptic. An agent destructive to germs.

GESUNDHEIT
A German word traditionally used to affirm the health of one who sneezes. Originally, it was said to prevent that person from sneezing his soul out and to drive away evil spirits that may have come out with the explosive breath.

GILL
Also quartern.

GINSENG

Also chin sang. An herbal remedy found in Asia and North America. It was believed to be a cure-all in colonial America. It grew wild in eastern North America and Native Americans used it for nausea and vomiting and as an ingredient in love potions and charms. The Chinese call it "the herb of eternal life" and have been using the herb since antiquity. In China, simply finding this plant is considered a good omen.

GLAIR

A mucoid, viscous discharge similar to an egg white.

GLANDERS

Also equinia, farcy. An infectious disease of horses and related animals communicable to humans and characterized by fever and inflammation of the skin and mucous membrane. It is called glanders proper when it affects the mucous membrane, particularly the nasal cavity where ulcers and abscesses are formed. This type often resulted in death. Farcy is the skin form of glanders, wherein farcy buds (nodules like those found in tuberculosis) are found on limbs, chest, and abdomen.

GLASS LEECH

Also doctor's sucking glass. An apparatus for drawing blood. It consisted of a tube of glass or metal used as a straw, which was attached to a container (often a small gourd) placed on the skin.

GLEET

Also gonorrhea.

GLISTER

Also clyster.

GODFREY'S CORDIAL

A patent remedy for infants, imported from Britain to "quiet the baby" in the 19th century. The principle ingredient was opium.

GOITER

Also struma.

GOLD

A metal used as a remedy for epilepsy, migraine, diabetes,

tuberculosis, syphilis, and alcoholism during the 19th and early 20th centuries. In the 17th century, alchemists claimed to be able to make a drinkable gold that could cure many diseases. It was often used when herbal remedies did not work.

GOLDENSEAL
Also yellow root.

GONORRHEA
Also clap, gleet. An infectious venereal disease characterized by an inflammation of the genitourinary tract resulting in painful urination and profuse discharge. Medically, the discharge was called "gleet," which later became a term to denote the disease itself.

GOOD MEDICINE
A Native American belief in the supernatural power of a person or thing to protect others.

GOOSE QUILL
The hollow shaft of the goose feather. When snipped at both ends, it was used to blow remedies into the body in the 17th and 18th centuries.

GOUT
A condition characterized by recurring sudden attacks of painful inflammation of the small joints, particularly, of the great toe. The attack usually occurred at night and disappeared with a sweat in the morning. In the 19th century it was believed to be common among "high livers." In the Middle ages it was believed to be caused by an unknown agent falling drop by drop into the joint.

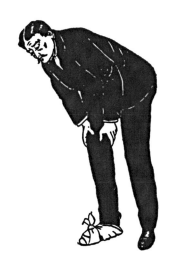

GRAHAMISM
A popular health system in the mid-19th century. Sylvester Graham, a physician who originated the system, attributed good

health to a vegetarian diet and the use of whole grain cereals. Graham bread and graham crackers came into the marketplace during that time.

GRANNY WOMAN
Also midwife.
And a woman who practiced folk medicine in Appalachia.

GRAPE CURE
A medical remedy for the treatment of pulmonary tuberculosis in the 19th and early 20th centuries. It consisted of the ingestion of large amounts of grapes.

GRAVE ROBBERS
Also sack-'em-up-men.

GREASELESS OINTMENT
Also vanishing cream.

GREASY PASTE
Also vernix. The natural thick, oily substance covering the body of the infant at birth.

GREAT LEPROSY
Also variola.

GREAT WHITE SCOURGE (THE)
Also tuberculosis.

GREEGREE
Also mojo.

GREEN SICKNESS
Also chlorosis.

GREEN WOUND
An infected wound that had a green-yellow discharge and a foul odor.

GRIP
Also influenza.

GRISGRIS [GRIGRI]
Also mojo.

GROCER'S ITCH
A condition of psoriasis or eczema of the hands of the grocer due to irritation from flour, sugar, and other items stocked in the store.

GROUND ITCH
Also dew itch, toe itch, water itch. A severe, itching inflammation of the skin of the feet caused by hookworm larvae burrowing through the skin.

GUM ARABIC
Also acacia. The viscous substance exuded by certain trees and shrubs native to Egypt. This substance was dried and used in medicine chiefly to relieve irritation from catarrhal affections of the mouth and throat. In the 19th century it was injected in solution into the veins for the treatment of hemorrhage and shock. Pharmaceutically it is still used for the formation of troches.

GUM BUSH
Also yerba santa.

GUM RASH
Also red gum.

HABITUAL FEVER
Also hectic fever.

HAMAMELIS WATER
Also witch hazel water. A remedy made from the bark of a shrub found in this country. Used externally as an application for bruises, headaches, and piles in the 19th and 20th centuries. Native Americans drank the tea as a tonic and as a rinse for throat irritations. The "regulars" frequently prescribed it as a gargle for sore throats in the 19th and early 20th centuries.

HAND

A unit of measure approximately equal to the breadth of a hand, about four inches.

HARELIP

A fissure of the upper lip noted at birth, it was split like a hare's.

HARTSHORN

Also ammonia water. A solution of ammonia, originally made from a decoction of the shaving's of a male deer's horn. It was used as a heart stimulant and an expectorant.

HASTY PUDDING

Also mush. A thick gruel made with cornmeal in America and often used as pap for infants. It was made with wheat grain in England and with oatmeal in Scotland.

HAWKER

Also drummer.

HAWKING

The noisy effort to raise mucous matter from the throat.

HAY ASTHMA

Also autumnal catarrh.

HAY FEVER

Also autumnal catarrh.

HEAD BATH

An intermittent soaking of the head in an herbal solution. Used as a treatment for deafness, loss of taste or smell, alcoholic poisoning, and inflammation of the brain.

HEAD LOUSE REMEDY

Also African American head louse remedy. In the 18th century, African Americans removed lice from their heads through this traditional treatment of plastering the hair with clay or earth, letting it dry, and then washing it with soap and water.

HEALTH BELT
A patent remedy for weak men in the 19th century. A belt of red flannel, which had wire attachments that made it appear electric, was worn next to the skin. It sent a burning sensation to the skin of the wearer which was caused not by an electrical current but by cayenne pepper impregnated into the red flannel.

HEBETUDE
A condition of unresponsiveness during serious fever states, characterized by a dullness of the senses and intellect.

HECTIC FEVER
Also habitual fever. A daily, recurring rise in temperature with accompanying chills, reddened cheeks, and sweat. It occurred in pulmonary tuberculosis and, sometimes, in septicemia.

HECTIC FLUSH
The reddened cheeks seen in hectic fever.

HELPER
Also herb.

HEMICRANIA
Also migraine.

HEPATITIS
Also liver complaint. An inflammation of the liver, generally characterized by jaundice, liver enlargement, fever, and malaise.

HERB
Also helper, yarb, yerb.
And a plant or plant part that has been used for remedies, nutritional additives, seasoning, or coloring.

HERBAL
Of or referring to herbs.
And a plant remedy book.

HERBALIST
A collector of herbs for botanical classification or remedial purposes.

And also Indian herbalist. A role assignment in some Native American tribes. This person did not possess the supernatural powers of the medicine man but had a knowledge of both good and bad medicine and sometimes acted as a sweat doctor.

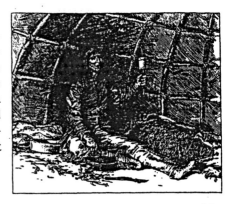

HEROIC THERAPY

A generic term for the methods of disease treatment espoused by the "regulars" in the 19th century, such as bloodletting, blistering and the use of purgatives and emetics. It was believed that these heroic therapies were most effective since the patient's response was very rapid and observable.

HERPES ZOSTER

Also shingles.

HESED

A Jewish term for an act of loving-kindness for another.

HEX

A curse, spell, or charm meant to hurt an individual or his property.

And a counter-charm to protect against sorcery.

HEXEDOKTOR [HEXERDOKTOR, HEXDOKTER]

A Pennsylvania German term for a professional powwower who achieved the status of "witch doctor" and was especially powerful in counter-charms against witchcraft. They were called upon mainly for the removal of spells cast by neighboring witches.

HICCOUGH [HICCUP, HICKET]

Also singultus. A convulsive catch in respiration caused by a spasm of the diaphragm. At times, continuous hiccoughs were a complication of influenza or encephalitis.

HIP

Also huckle. The joint between thigh bone and pelvic bone.

And the rounded area on the side of the body between the thigh and the waist.

HIP BATH
Also sitz bath. A bath in which the patient sits in the tub, bathing only the hips and buttocks.

HIPPOCRATES
A Greek physician born c. 460 B.C. and called the "Father of Medicine." He originated and taught the humoral theory of disease which was based on the belief that the body contains four humors: blood, phlegm, yellow bile, and black bile. A correct proportion or mixing of these humors constituted health. Incorrect proportion or irregular distribution constituted illness.

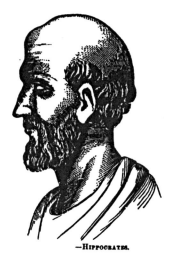

—HIPPOCRATES.

HIPPOPOTAMUS IVORY
The material that was used to make false teeth in the early 1800s.

HIVES
Also nettle rash, urticaria. A condition characterized by skin eruptions and severe itching. The causes were believed to be multiple, including gastrointestinal disorders and menstruation.

And, in England in the 19th century, a term applied to croup, laryngitis, and chicken pox.

HIVE SYRUP
Also squill syrup. A syrup made using the root of the squill plant and believed to be a remedy for croup and bronchitis.

HOGSHEAD [HOGSHED]
A large barrel holding up to 140 gallons and used to carry liquids, e.g., water or wine, to customers. Water was delivered house to house in large cities in America, and wine was transported to hotels and taverns through the 19th century.

HOLY HERB
Also yerba santa.

HOLY WATER
Water blessed by a Catholic priest.
And a Native American word for whiskey in the 1800s.

HOMEOPATHY
A system of disease treatment based on two beliefs: one, that diseases are cured by the administration of drugs which produce effects on the body similar to the symptoms of the disease; and two, that the smaller the dose given the more powerful the effect of the drug. This system was created by Dr. Samuel Hahnemann in the early 19th century. Compare **ALLOPATHY**.

HOME REMEDIES
Medical treatments (generally, herbal remedies) passed down in families from generation to generation.

HOMOSEXUAL
Also urning.

HOODOO DOCTOR
Also voodoo doctor.

HOOKWORM DISEASE
Also ancylostomiasis, dochmiasis, Egyptian chlorosis, lazyworm disease, miner's disease, St. Gotthard's tunnel disease, tunnel anemia, uncinariasis. It was a world-wide condition caused by a parasite that entered the body, usually, through the skin of the feet and ankles and attached itself to the intestine causing a state of anemia, physical deterioration, and mental fatigue. The cause was discovered in the 1880s and treatment consisted of essence of thyme (thymol), three drops, followed with Epsom salts.

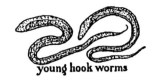

young hook worms

Much enlarged.

HOOPEN COUGH [HOOPING COUGH]
Also whooping cough.

HOPS

The fruit of a plant native to North America and Europe.

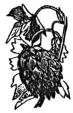

Hop.

And an herbal remedy that has been used for many illnesses, particularly, digestive disorders. Application of a hops poultice to the body was used to increase healing locally. Sleeping on a pillow of hops was believed to produce a sedative effect.

HORSE COLD

Also autumnal catarrh.

HOSPITAL GANGRENE

Also St. Anthony's fire. A suppurative inflammation in the wounds of individuals in military hospitals. It was fatal and believed to be contagious.

HOT BATH

A water bath treatment in which the water temperature ranged from 104° to 110° Fahrenheit and was followed by a cold bath and a rubdown. Its expected action was to stimulate the nervous system by producing perspiration and increasing pulse and respiration.

HOUNGAN

Also boco, boko. A voodoo cult priest that read the future regarding health and food supplies through shells, small sticks, or ashes.

HOUSEMAID'S KNEE

A chronic inflammation and swelling of the small fluid-filled sac in the front of the kneecap. It was believed to be caused by long-term trauma to the knee.

HUCKLE

Also hip.

HUMBUG

Also buncombe.

HUMOR [HUMOUR]
Any fluid or semifluid of the body.

And one of the four health-influencing fluids of the body as defined by Hippocrates: yellow bile, black bile, phlegm, and blood. See **HIPPOCRATES.**

And a disposition of temperament, as Galen's humors: choleric, melancholic, phlegmatic, and sanguine. See **GALEN.**

And a chronic, moist skin disease.

HUNGER CURE
Treatment of disease by fasting.

HYDRARGYRUM
Also mercury.

HYDROCEPHALUS
Also water head, water on the brain. An abnormal collection of body fluids in the fluid holding chambers (ventricles) of the cranium. It is usually found in newborns and noted by eventual enlargement of the head, mental impairment, and convulsions.

HYDRONE
The water molecule, H_2O.

HYDRONICK
Also watery. The process of giving off a water-like substance.

HYDROPATHY
The use of water in the treatment and cure of all diseases by the "irregulars."

HYDROPHOBIA
Also rabies.

And a morbid fear of water. This fear, it was believed, was the reason individuals affected by rabies resisted taking water and other fluids. Later it was found that water and fluids were refused due to an inability to swallow caused by the disease.

HYDROPS [HYDROPSY]
Also dropsy.

HYDROPS ASCITES
Also abdominal dropsy.

HYDROTHERAPY
Also Kneipp cure. The treatment of disease by application of water in various forms and temperatures by the "regulars." According to Kneipp therapy, wading through wet, dewy grass was especially beneficial.

HYDROTHORAX
Also dropsy of the chest. The presence of fluid in the chest.

HYPNOTISM
Also animal magnetism.

HYSTERIA
A nervous condition that occurred episodically and simulated signs and symptoms of other diseases. It was most commonly found in young women. In the Middle Ages it was believed to be caused by the uterus.

ICTERIC
A remedy for jaundice.
And pertaining to or characterized by jaundice.

ICTERITIOUS
Also jaundiced. Having a yellow or yellowish color, especially of the skin, as occurs in jaundice.

IMMUNITY
The condition of the body that enables it to resist disease.

IMMUNIZATION
Also passive immunization. The process of rendering a subject resistant to a disease by injection of serum from animals that have developed resistance to the disease.

And also active immunization. The process of rendering a subject resistant to disease by inoculation or vaccination. The first immunization was against smallpox. See **INOCULATION** and **VACCINATION**.

IMPERIAL
A home remedy made up of cream of tartar and sugar. Served cool to those with fevers.

IMPETIGO
Also scrum pox.

INANITION
The wasting of the body from starvation.

INCANTATION
The singing of special words or a magic formula in casting a counterspell to remove illness from the body of the patient.

INCONTINENCE
The inability to control the escape of bodily discharges, particularly feces and/or urine.

INCUBUS
Also nightmare, nocturnal asthma. A frightening dream accompanied with pressure on the chest and a feeling of powerlessness to move or speak.

And, in the belief of the Middle Ages, a male demon supposed to have sexual connection with women in their sleep.

INDIAN BALM
Also birthroot.

INDIAN DREAM FULFILLMENT
Also dream fulfillment.

INDIAN ENEMA
Also enema.

INDIAN GUM
Also ragged cup, rosin weed, silphium. A plant used by Native

Americans and European Americans to make a gum that was chewed to cleanse their teeth and sweeten their breath.

INDIAN HERBALIST
Also herbalist.

INDIAN MAGIC MEDICINE
The practice of preventing and curing disease mainly using charms, dances, and song. Tricks were part of the practice. Sleight of hand maneuvers were used to remove offending objects perceived to be the immediate cause of an illness. The shaman would place his hand over or on the body of the ill person and appear to remove the cause of the illness, perhaps a stone or other small object. The hand that had held nothing suddenly held the offending object. The juggler's lodge was another example of the shaman's magical power to communicate with supernatural forces to help supplicants.

INDIAN MAGIC MEDICINE STONE
Also magic medicine stone.

INDIAN MAGIC NUMBERS
Also magic numbers.

INDIAN MEDICINE ARROW
Also medicine arrow.

INDIAN MEDICINE BAG
Also medicine bag.

INDIAN MEDICINE DANCE
Also medicine dance.

INDIAN MEDICINE HAT
Also medicine hat.

INDIAN MEDICINE PIPE
Also medicine pipe.

INDIAN MEDICINE RATTLE
Also medicine rattle.

INDIAN MEDICINE SONG
Also medicine song.

INDIAN PINK
Also pinkroot.

INDIAN SAGE
Also boneset.

INDIAN SMOKE TREATMENT
Also smoke treatment.

INDIAN SWEAT BATH
Also sweat bath.

INDIAN SWEAT DOCTOR
Also sweat doctor.

INDIAN SWEAT LODGE
Also sweat lodge.

INDIAN TOBACCO
Also pukeweed.

INDIAN WITCHCRAFT
Also witchcraft.

INDIFFERENT BATH
A treatment using tepid water. Believed to produce a sedative effect.

INFANTILE ATROPHY
Also marasmus.

INFANTILE DIARRHEA
Also cholera infantum.

INFANTILE ECLAMPSIA
Also tooth spasm. A convulsion of childhood. It was often attributed to teething and the accompanying fever. Death was a frequent result.

INFECTIOUS

Capable of or easily communicating a disease.

INFECTIOUS DISEASE

An illness caused by microorganisms or germs, which are capable of multiplication in the body where they produce poisons that cause the symptoms of the illness. Most diseases are infectious, though not necessarily contagious. Others, e.g. scabies, are contagious but not infectious.

INFLAMMATION

Also phlogosis.

INFLUENZA

Also epidemic catarrh, grip, la grippe, lightning catarrh. An acute, infectious disease that attacks one of three systems: respiratory, gastrointestinal, or nervous. It is characterized by fever, inflammation of mucous membranes with discharge, pain in muscles, and rapid exhaustion. The most common complications in the 19th and early 20th centuries were pneumonia and, occasionally, insanity.

And Spanish influenza, the name given to the pandemic of an acute influenza-like disease which was found in Europe and America during the summer and autumn of 1918.

INFUSION

The steeping of a medicinal plant in cold or hot water to make a tea.

INHALATION OF GAS

A form of pneumotherapy. Inhalations of carbonic acid and sulfurous acid were used to treat tuberculosis of the lungs, asthma, and emphysema.

INNUTRITION

A lack of food and/or a problem in the process by which food builds and repairs tissue in the body.

INOCULATION

Also engrafting. The insertion of a contagium into the tissues of living plants or animals or into culture mediums for the purpose of study.

And also buying the disease, preventive inoculation. The insertion of a contagium into a body for the purpose of producing a mild form of a disease, which would be severe if contracted in the usual way. This procedure was used in ancient China to prevent smallpox: dried smallpox scabs were stuffed into the nose of a child (left nostril for boys; right for girls). In Europe and the American colonies in the early 1700s, needles bathed in smallpox pus were used to introduce the contagium into the body. Although inoculation was believed by some to be contrary to the will of God, it became fairly well accepted practice by the late 1700s and was given on a large scale in the cities of the United States. See **IMMUNIZATION** and **VACCINATION**.

INSANITY
Also madness.

INSECTS
Also bugs.

INSOLATION
A treatment using exposure to the sun's rays, a sun bath.
And sunstroke.

INTERMITTENT FEVER
Also malaria.
And an attack of fever that is broken up into regular recurring events separated by periods of normal temperature.

INVALID
Also valetudinarian. A person chronically ill and/or disabled.

INVOLUNTARY [AN]
Stool discharged due to an episode of bowel incontinence.

IPECAC
The dried root of a shrub native to South America. In large doses it acts as an emetic, and in small doses it causes sweating, brings about coughing needed to remove phlegm from the lungs, and stimulates digestion. In the 19th century, it was used as an emetic for adults with narcotic poisoning, and for children with croup it was used to help dislodge the membranes and secretions that interfered with breathing. It is a specific drug for amebic dysentery.

IRONING TREATMENT
Also Chinese ironing treatment.

IRREGULAR AGUE
Also dumb ague.

IRREGULARS
A term most often used by the "regulars" for individuals who practiced medicine without the benefit of a medical school education.

ISCHEMIA
See **ANEMIA.**

ISSUE
A small wound artificially produced with a caustic or a knife, into which a pellet of wood or root or a twisted strip of cloth (seton) was inserted to maintain drainage.

ITCH (THE)
Also la galle, prairie itch, scabies. A contagious skin disease caused by the burrowing of a mite under the skin characterized by intense itching and subsequent eczema. It was very common in the Middle Ages and continued to be a problem through the 19th century.

JAIL FEVER
Also typhus.

JALAP
Also man root. A type of plant used by Native Americans as a remedy for many different illnesses. Spanish colonizers used a Mexican variety as a purgative. The "regulars" also used it for its powerful purgative effects.
And also May apple.

JAMESTOWN WEED
Also jimsonweed.

JAPANESE AMERICAN PREGNANCY TABOO
The belief that dark animals should not be kept as pets in the home of a pregnant woman or the baby would be born with a very dark complexion.

JAUNDICE
A condition caused by the presence of bile and characterized by the yellow appearance of the skin, mucous membranes, and body secretions.

JAUNDICED
Also icteritious.

JENNER, EDWARD
The physician that introduced the vaccination against smallpox in 1796.

JERKS (THE)
A contagious condition occurring in individuals during religious camp meetings in Kentucky. Characterized by violent shaking in every joint to the point of falling down.

JESUITS' BARK
Also cinchona bark, Peruvian bark. A remedy used by Native South Americans for fevers. Settlers adopted it for use as an anti-malarial remedy after 1630. Quinine was found to be the active element in the bark in 1819, and by the mid-1800s quinine was available for use as an antipyretic.

JIGGER
Also chigger, chigoe, flea, pulex. A parasitic insect that lives on the skin of humans and animals.

JIMSONWEED
Also angel's trumpet, Jamestown weed, stinkweed, thorn apple. An herb whose leaves were smoked to relieve bronchial and asthmatic conditions. Although Native Americans used the seeds to induce visions and for poultices applied to burns and

inflammations, it is not certain if the plant is native to North America. In the early 1900s an American pharmaceutical company used it to produce atropine, a drug frequently used in the practice of medicine.

JOHNNY APPLESEED
A legendary figure known for distribution of apple seeds in the late 1700s. He also was a preacher and a healer. He shared many medicinal herbs, especially mayweed, which he believed to be a cure for malaria. Native Americans believed him to be a great medicine man.

JOINT OIL
Also synovial fluid. The viscous fluid found in joint cavities.

JOURNEY PROUD
A temporary change of demeanor prior to beginning a trip. Characterized by a kind of excitement and sometimes accompanied by a loss of appetite and/or sleeplessness.

JUGGLER
Also medicine man.

And a Native American who used sleight of hand to provide observers with performances supposedly reflecting powers of healing skill.

JUGGLER'S LODGE
A cylindrical enclosure made by planting four or more poles and wrapping them with sheets of bark, skins or blankets to serve as a covering wherein the medicine man communicated with the spirits to obtain knowledge of future events. When the medicine man concealed himself inside the structure, it swayed violently from side to side while loud thumping noises and voices were heard from within. Seemingly, the medicine man was communicating with the spirits. Questions were put to the medicine man, and answers were given. This "magic" act became more mysterious with its retelling by European Americans. In their version the medicine man was tied up with a rope and carried into the structure; upon opening the structure after the ritual the rope was gone, but it would be found in some other part of the village.

JUMPER

An individual with a nervous disorder characterized by a sudden jump or violent movement when touched or addressed suddenly in a loud voice. A medical term used through the mid-1900s.

KAFFEE

Also coffee.

KERMES

A type of insect, often found in oak trees, whose dried bodies were used to make a red dye.

KEROSENE

Also coal oil, lamp oil. A petroleum product commonly used as an illuminating oil. It was used externally as a remedy for lung problems, diseases of the skin and paralysis. Internally, it has been used for tapeworm infestation.

KICKAPOO COUGH SYRUP

A patent remedy made up of rum and molasses. This 19th century nostrum sold well due to the then popular belief in the efficacy of Native American medicine. The name was designed to sound Indian-like in order to help sales.

KIDNEY

Also rein, ren. Either of the two urine-producing glands, found in the loins.

KIDNEY DISEASE

Also Bright's disease.

KILLED MERCURY

Mercury which has lost its fluidity through mixing with lemon juice or turpentine.

KINDLING FOODS

Foods that help other foods to burn efficiently as fuel for the body. At the same time kindling foods supply their own elements which the body needs. Vegetables and fruits, other than potatoes, peas and beans, are examples. This term was used in the early 20th century.

KING'S EVIL

Also scrofula.

KNEIPP CURE

Also hydrotherapy.

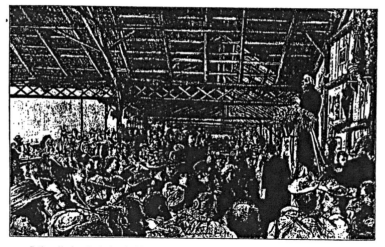

Father Kneipp Lecturing to his Patients on the Natural Method of Living and Healing.

KOLA NUT

Also cola nut. The seed of the kola tree. Originally used as a stimulant and a substitute for tea and coffee in Africa.

KOPP'S BABY FRIEND

A patent medicine used as a sedative for infants. The principle ingredient was morphine. Late 1800s.

KOPF TETTER [KOPP TETTER]

A Pennsylvania German remedy for dandruff. It consisted of sage or burdock leaves.

KUGELFEST

Also stab-frees, stick-frees. The Pennsylvania German use of the power of the charm to make an individual bulletproof.

KÜMMEL

A liquor flavored with caraway oil. Used as a digestive stimulant and to reduce gas and colic.

LACTOSE

Also milk sugar.

LADY WEBSTER'S PILLS

A patent remedy used as a laxative. The principle ingredient was aloe.

LA GALLE [LA GALE]

Also itch.

LA GRIPPE

Also influenza.

LAMP OIL

Also kerosene.

LANCET

Also physician's pocket companion. A small, pointed and two-edged surgical knife.

LANCET RING

A ring worn on the finger of the surgeon that contained a hidden curved blade used to pierce the skin of the patient.

LARD

Also adeps. The purified internal fat of the abdomen of the hog. Used in remedies as a basis for ointments.

LARYNGEAL DIPHTHERIA
Also diphtheritic croup.

LARYNGEAL STRIDOR
Also child-crowing.

LASK
Also scouring.

LATENT AGUE
Also dumb ague.

LAUDABLE PUS
A creamy, yellowish, odorless discharge from inflamed tissue believed to be essential to the healing of wounds.

LAUGHING GAS
Also nitrous oxide. A pleasant-smelling general anesthetic used by dentists for short procedures. Some patients would react with laughter and exhilaration after inhaling the gas.

LAZYWORM DISEASE
Also hookworm disease.

LEAD COLIC
Also painter's colic.

LEADEN BULLETS
Swallowed as a medical treatment for spasms of the intestines, called "twisting of the guts," in the early 18th century. See **COLIC**.

LEECH
Also bloodsucker. A bloodsucking worm used for the local abstraction of blood. Each leech could draw from one-half to one ounce of blood when placed on the body of the patient. Leeches would loosen their hold after an application of table salt.
And a common name for a doctor prior to the 20th century.

LEECHING
A once highly esteemed therapeutic measure in which a blood-sucking worm or a cupping glass was applied to the body. It was a

very common practice, up to the middle of the 20th century, in the management of acute affections of the eye, ear, and, occasionally, of the coverings of the lungs and abdominal organs.

LEPRA
Also leprosy. A chronic, infectious disease endemic in tropical and subtropical regions characterized by skin and subcutaneous tissue destruction. It was known in Biblical times when it was not differentiated from conditions such as psoriasis, vitiligo, and albinism.

LEPROSY
Also lepra.

LEUCORRHEA [LEUKORRHEA]
Also the whites.

LICE
Plural of louse.

LIEN
Also spleen.

LIGHT AND AIR BATHS
A treatment that exposed the naked body to sun and air. Usually practiced in special huts or cottages.

LIGHTNING CATARRH
Also influenza.

LIME WATER
Also liquor calcis. A solution of lime diluted with water. Used as a remedy for vomiting and indigestion and taken in amounts of one-half to two ounces.

LIMEY
A nickname for the British sailor after 1795. It was then that each sailor began to receive a daily ration of lemon or lime to prevent scurvy.

LIQUOR CALCIS
Also lime water.

LISK
Also loin.

LISTERISM
The practice of asepsis according to the principles of Dr. Joseph Lister. Carbolic acid was used to kill germs and maintain an antiseptic environment in the surgery, during the surgical process, and in the dressings used to cover surgical wounds. Late 19th century.

LITTLE APPLE
Also camomile.

LIVER COMPLAINT
Also hepatitis.

LOBELIA
Also pukeweed.

LOCAL ANEMIA
See **ANEMIA.**

LOCKJAW
Also tetanus.

LOIN
Also lisk. That part of the side and back of the body between the ribs and pelvis.
And **LOINS.** Also lisk. That part of the hip and lower abdomen believed in antiquity to be the region of strength and procreative powers.

LOMBARDY LEPROSY
Also pellagra.

LONG IN THE TOOTH
Having attained old age.

LOUSE
Also pediculus. A small parasitic insect that affects the skin. There are three common varieties, named according to where they

live on the body: the body louse, the head louse and the pubic louse (crab louse).

LOUSE TYPHUS
Also typhus.

LOUSY
Infested with lice.

LOVE APPLE
Also tomato.

LOZENGE
Also troche.

LUES
Also syphilis.

LULAV
A Jewish term for a palm frond originally used in an ancient harvest ritual to summon the wind gods to bless the harvest and prevent famine. The palm frond has since been adopted to symbolize agricultural origins during the Jewish harvest festival of thanksgiving.

LUMBAGO
Also backache. A rheumatic condition of the lower back characterized by pain and rigidity.

LUNACY
Also madness.

LYDIA E. PINKHAM'S VEGETABLE COMPOUND FOR WOMEN
A patent medicine for female problems. It contained 18% alcohol as well as vegetable teas.

LYMPHATIC TEMPERAMENT
Also phlegmatic temperament.

LYSSA
Also rabies.

MACFADDEN, BERNARR [MCFADDEN, BERNARD]

A health reformer of the early to mid-1900s. He was a naturopath who believed that disease could be prevented by vigorous exercise and "good food." "Good food" included fresh fruits, vegetables, and whole wheat bread. Coffee, tea, alcohol, and drugs of all kinds were to be avoided. Disease was treated by fasting. He was strongly critical of traditional medicine of his day and recommended that physicians teach people to avoid illness.

MADNESS

Also craziness, insanity, lunacy, moonstruck. An acquired, chronic condition of the mind characterized by change of character and habit, marked by delusions, illusions, or hallucinations.

And a derangement of intellect.

And the condition of being of unsound mind.

MADONNA WORSHIP

Italian Americans paid tribute to the healing powers of the Virgin Mary (Madonna) on festival days. Worshipers brought wax images of legs, arms, hearts and candles with pictures to appeal to the Madonna for healing and/or continued well-being.

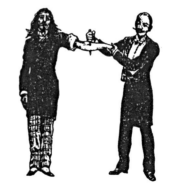

MAGICIAN

Also medicine man.

And someone who uses charms, spells, and rituals to appear to control events.

MAGIC MEDICINE

The ancient art or practice of preventing and curing disease with the aid of supernatural forces, which were called upon through objects such as amulets and rituals such as ceremonial dances. See also **INDIAN MAGIC MEDICINE**.

MAGIC MEDICINE STONE

Also Indian magic medicine stone. A special stone used by the medicine man and believed to be a very strong remedy capable of removing a spell or counteracting a poison. It was rubbed on a wound, or scrapings were made into a tea for drinking.

MAGIC NUMBERS

Also Indian magic numbers. Native Americans believed the numbers four and six to be sacred as they symbolized the four directions plus the northeast/west and southeast/west parameters. One way of using the power of these numbers was to incorporate them into healing rituals. For example treatments and/or remedies would be repeated four or six times.

MAGIC PICTURE

A Navajo Indian remedy for treating illnesses. They create an intricate design with sand which makes their Holy People visible. The patient may sit on the design to seek healing. At sunset the design is scattered to prevent evil spirits from coming and making mischief.

MAIMONIDES, MOSES

A medieval Spanish rabbinic philosopher and physician who believed that the preservation of health and life was a divine commandment. Among his many writings were several medical books, the most popular being *Regimen of Health*, which includes the concept of "a healthy mind in a healthy body."

MALARIA

Also ague, ager, estivoautumnal fever, fever and ague, intermittent fever, malarial fever, marsh fever, miasmatic fever, paludism, periodic fever, remittent fever. An acute and sometimes chronic, infectious, febrile disease transmitted by the bite of the mosquito. It is characterized by attacks of chills and fever and sweating. It was described in the time of Hippocrates.

MALARIAL FEVER

Also malaria.

MALAXATION

A kneading motion in the art of massage.

MAL D'ESTOMAC
Also dirt eating.

MAL FRANÇAISE
Also syphilis.

MALIGNANT EDEMA
Also gangrenous emphysema, gas gangrene. The swelling of tissue following an injury caused by gas forming microbes in the damaged tissue. The swelling extends rapidly and destroys tissue. It had an extremely high mortality rate.

And a form of anthrax in which the head, neck and arms have marked swelling and blisters which tended to become gangrenous.

MALIGNANT SORE THROAT
Also septic sore throat. A severe inflammation of the posterior portion of the mouth (pharynx) and tonsils believed to be caused by an unclean milk supply.

MALJO
An African American belief. If a person with a "bad eye" looks at a child and comments on his/her beauty the child will become sick, that is, gets maljo. It is similar to the Greek American concept of the "evil eye."

MALT
A grain, such as barley, maize, rye, or wheat, which has been made to germinate and then baked to dry. Used as a nutrient to treat wasting diseases.

MAMBO
A female Voodoo cult leader.

MAMMA
Also breast, mammary gland. The milk secreting organ of the mother.

MAMMARY GLAND
Also mamma.

MAN MIDWIFE
A physician that offered his services to replace the midwife in the mid-1700s.

MAN ROOT
Also jalap, Satan's apple.

MANZANILLA
Also camomile.

MARASMUS
Also infantile atrophy. Extreme wasting that occurred in newborns and young children without obvious cause.

MARASMUS SENILIS
Also senile atrophy. A condition characterized by the gradual wasting of the body in those of advanced age.

MARSH FEVER
Also malaria.

MARSH MIASMA
A vaporous substance believed to rise from stagnant water or putrid matter and to float in the air, especially at night, like a poisonous gas.

MASKED AGUE
Also dumb ague.

MATRON
A female superintendent in a public institution, usually a hospital or prison.

MATTER
A discharge, often purulent, from diseased tissue.

MAW
Also stomach, ventriculus. A sac-like cavity in human beings and other animals for holding and digesting food.

MAY APPLE
Also American mandrake, duck's foot, jalap, wild lemon. A plant

used by Native Americans to induce vomiting and as a laxative. European Americans used it to treat multiple illnesses. It has no relation to the European mandrake.

MAYIDISM [MAYIDISMUS]
Also pellagra.

MAYWEED
Also camomile.

MEAD
An alcoholic liquor made of fermented honey and malt; spices were added for flavor.
And a soft drink made of sirup of sarsaparilla and carbonated water.

MEAL
Edible grains, e.g., wheat and rye, coarsely ground.

MEASLES
Also morbilli. An acute, infectious disease characterized by chills, fever, cough, catarrhal inflammation of the air ways and the eyes, and a skin rash appearing about four days after the fever. The disease is very contagious and affects chiefly children. Common complications were ear infections, pneumonia, bronchitis, and tuberculosis.

MEDICATED WINES
Pharmaceutic menstruums using wine as a base.

MEDICINE
The science of the treatment of disease.
And any substance given for the cure of disease.

MEDICINE ARROW
Also Indian medicine arrow. A special arrow that was part of the healing ceremony of some Native American tribes. It was believed that the power of the medicine man could be increased by calling up animal spirits by means of the arrow. The arrow would catch the disease of the patient and then be taken to a deep pit and destroyed.

MEDICINE BAG

Also bundle, Indian medicine bag, pouch. A Native American container made from the skin of an animal. It contained herbs, roots, and sacred objects and was worn attached to the clothing of its owner. Believed to have great protective and mystic powers, it was often passed on through generations of the same family.

MEDICINE DANCE

Also Indian medicine dance. A general term that included many Native American ceremonies relevant to tribal practices of medicine, culture, and religion.

MEDICINE HAT

Also Indian medicine hat. A head covering made and blest by a Native American medicine man and worn on special occasions by those granted and/or claiming some healing art skill.

MEDICINE MAN

Also conjurer, juggler, magician, physician, priest, shaman, theurgist, trickster. (This multiplicity of terms used by European Americans to identify the medicine man reflects the wide variety of perceptions to the Native Americans' healing arts.) A Native American whose chief functions were to treat the sick, and take preventive measures against sickness, drought, food shortage, and enemy raids. They based their treatments in the power of charms, prayers, and rituals to drive evil spirits away.

And see **CHINESE MEDICINE MEN.**

MEDICINE PIPE

Also Indian medicine pipe. A ceremonial pipe of Native American plains tribes. Decorated with feathers, skins, and painted designs, it could only be touched by the medicine man and was used in ceremonies to treat the sick and guard the tribe from harm. When it was not being used in ceremonies it was kept wrapped in a bundle in the home of the medicine man. According to some historians, the medicine pipe was never smoked; others say it was smoked at designated times during a ceremony.

MEDICINE PIPE BUNDLE

A special bag used by some Native American tribes to hold their medicine pipe. It was opened during their annual sacred cereemonies when they gathered in the Holy Tipi. The pipe was believed to be all powerful and thought to protect all the members of the tribe.

MEDICINE RATTLE

Also Indian medicine rattle. Usually, a hollow gourd with loose seeds inside used by Native American healers in treating the sick. It was believed that the noise would drive away evil spirits.

MEDICINE SHOWS

Traveling entertainment provided for country people by vendors of patent medicine. Native Americans were brought along as part of the entertainment to authenticate the value of the "Indian" remedies being sold as cure-alls. They operated from the 18th century until World War I.

MEDICINE SONG

Also Indian medicine song. A unique prayer song directed to the Great Spirit or Creator and sung by the Native American medicine man or other assigned tribal member when sickness occurred. Believed to impact indirectly on the patient.

MEDICINE WOMAN

Native American women who practiced as healers. The assigned role varied from tribe to tribe. Medicine women of the Blackfoot tribe had a leading role in preparatory activities for the medicine dance. They initiated the sacred rite by praying for the welfare of the tribe, and then they erected the center pole of the medicine lodge in which the dance would take place. Their participation ended at this time. Women of the Ojibwa tribe also had an assisting role in rituals. They treated women and children for illness, and tattooed any member of the tribe for the cure of headache, toothache, and chronic neuralgia.

MEDIEVAL TIMES

Also Middle Ages.

MEGRIM

Also migraine.

MELANCHOLIA

Also climacteric insanity.

MELANCHOLIC TEMPERAMENT
A name for the disposition of one who is intellectual and well-spoken with a tendency to be irritable and depressed in spirit. See GALEN.

MELANCHOLY [MELANCHOLER]
Also black bile.

MEMBRANOUS ANGINA
Also diphtheria.

MEMBRANOUS CROUP
Also diphtheritic croup.

MENINGITIS
An epidemic cerebral spinal fever in which there is an inflammation of the covering of the brain and spinal cord. It was first described in a small outbreak in Geneva in 1805. Later there were serious outbreaks in America and in Europe. The mortality rate was over 70%.

MENSES
Also courses.

MENSTRUUM
A generic term for a solvent, a fluid containing another substance in solution. It is a very old term and is believed to be so named due to the alchemist's belief in the influence of the moon in dissolving solids.

MENTAGRA
Also sycosis.

MENTHA
Also mint.

MERCUROUS CHLORIDE [MERCUROUS CHLORID]
Also calomel.

MERCURY
Also hydrargyrum, quicksilver. It is a metallic element that was

used in remedies for internal and external treatments of multiple diseases and as an alterative.

MESCAL BUTTON
Also peyote.

MESMERISM
Also animal magnetism.

METAL FUME FEVER
Also brass founder's ague, spelter shakes, zinc fume fever. A condition occurring in those who were exposed to vapors of volatile metals. Characterized by symptoms similar to malaria.

METALLOTHERAPY
The treatment of disease by the application of metals to the skin. Metal disks or coins were placed or bandaged around the part to be acted on. Results were said to follow quickly. It was frequently used in cases of hysteria.

METEORISM
Also tympanites. The distention of the abdomen with gas.

METRIA
Pelvic inflammation after childbirth.

METRITIS
Inflammation of the womb (uterus).

MIASMA [MIASM]
Infectious material floating in the air arising from decomposing animal or vegetable matter.

MIASMATIC FEVER
Also malaria.

MICROBE
A generic term for minute organisms seen only under the microscope and believed to be the cause of disease. Late 19th century.

And germ, a bacteria (a specific kind of microorganism) that caused disease.

MICROBE KILLER

A patent remedy advertised as a cure-all in the late 19th century reflecting the historic discovery of microbes. It contained water with small amounts of red wine, hydrochloric acid, and sulfuric acid.

MIDDLE AGES

Also medieval times. The period of European history between c. 500 A.D. and 1450 A.D.

MIDEWIWIN [MIDE]

The Medicine Lodge Society of the Ojibwa Native American tribe. The lodge taught herbal lore, ethical behavior, and respect of the spirits. Women and men were members of the lodge, and they believed that the first Native American was a woman.

MIDWIFE

Also granny woman. A woman, with or without formal education, who assists in childbirth. It has been a woman's role since antiquity, passed along through female family members or assigned to a woman by the community. Formal education began in Europe in the mid-1700s for midwives and physicians.

And a female nurse who attends women in childbirth.

And, in the 19th century, a female obstetrician.

MIGRAINE

Also hemicrania, megrim, sick headache. A nervous condition characterized by a periodic headache, frequently on one side, and accompanied by nausea, vomiting, and vision and hearing disturbances.

MILIARIA

Also sweating disease.

MILK CRUST

Also tetter.

MILK FEVER

A condition characterized by a slight rise of temperature and hardening of the breasts of the mother after child-birth. Believed by some to be due to the formation of milk in the breasts, and believed by others to be a mild form of puerperal fever.

MILK SICKNESS

Also puking fever, sick stomach, the slows, the trembles. A disease of cattle communicated to people who drink their milk or eat their meat. Characterized by chills, vomiting, trembling, and disorders of the gastrointestinal system. A mysterious illness in the mid-1800s, it was later discovered to be caused in the cattle by ingestion of the white snake-root plant.

MILK SUGAR

Also lactose. A sweet carbohydrate found in the milk of mammals. It was used as a medium, to give bulk and sweetness, in the administration of medicine.

MILK TRANSFUSION

A treatment that consisted of an injection of 4 to 6 ounces of milk into a vein of the patient. Given for cholera collapse and traumatic hemorrhage.

MILKWORT

Also snakeroot.

MILLENIUM [MILLENNIUM]

A thousand years.

MILLER'S ASTHMA

Also autumnal catarrh.

MILT

Also spleen.

MINER'S DISEASE

Also hookworm disease.

MINT

Also mentha. An herb that became an important remedy in the 18th century. Peppermint and spearmint teas were used for headaches and a variety of gastrointestinal problems. They were used as a sedative and to treat hysteria by healers in the South. It was used as a substitute for coffee or regular tea.

MITE
Also tick. A minute, parasitic animal, related to the spider, that lives on the skin of humans and animals and transmits disease.

MITY
Infested with mites.

MOJO
Also greegree, grigri, grisgris. An African American charm bag which effected cures on those that carried it on their person. A more powerful type could let its possessor turn into an animal. The higher the price paid for the charm, the greater the power.

MOLASSES
Also treacle. A sweet, syrupy liquid left after the refining of sugar. Believed to be effective for catarrhal problems, and used for making of pills.

MOLIMENA [MOLIMINA]
Unpleasant symptoms, such as headache and malaise, accompanying menstrual periods.

MOON BLINDNESS
A condition of dimmed vision believed to be due to exposure of the eyes to moonlight when asleep.

MOONSHINE
Also tombstone hootch, wood alcohol, wood spirit. Illicit whiskey that can cause poisoning. Permanent blindness was a frequent complication in survivors. It was produced in America during the Prohibition era in the 1920s and believed to be produced in the foothills of Kentucky on a continuing basis.

MOONSTRUCK
Also madness.

MOON THERAPY
Also Chinese moon therapy.

MORBID
Of or related to a state of disease.

MORBID VIGILANCE
Also coma vigil, morbid wakefulness. A comatose condition in which a person's eyes remain open despite being unconscious and/or delirious.

MORBID WAKEFULNESS
Also morbid vigilance.

MORBILLI
Also measles.

MORBUS GALLICUS
Also syphilis.

MORIA
A type of dementia characterized by excessive, fatuous verbal expressions and an inability to be serious.

MORPHINISM
The morphine habit, an addiction.

MORTAR AND PESTLE
The device used by apothecaries to powder drugs to facilitate administration. The mortar is a hard bowl and the pestle is the instrument used to pound and grind the drug in the mortar. It became the symbol of the pharmacist.

MOTHER
Also womb.
And female parent.

MOTHER'S MARK
A colored patch of skin found on the body of a newborn--a birthmark.

MOUNTAIN BALM
Also yerba santa.

MOUNTAIN BOX
Also bearberry.

MOUNTAIN FLAX
Also snakeroot.

MOUTH BADNESS
Also scurvy.

MOUTH ROT
Also trench mouth.

MOXA
A coil of cotton, treated so as to burn slowly, which was ignited and placed on the skin as a counterirritant. It was a part of Eastern and Western medicine through the 20th century.

MOXIBUSTION
An ancient traditional Chinese treatment in which acupuncture points were treated with hot or glowing medicinal herbs to ease rheumatic pains. Sometimes hot iron rods were used. In the early 20th century, direct contact with the herb was not required. The herb was wrapped in a paper to be held over the body while burning, or made into the shape of a ball or cone to be placed on the body and removed before it burned the patient.

MUCOUS MEMBRANE
The lining of those cavities of the body that communicate with the air and secrete mucus.

MUCUS
The sticky, watery secretion that covers mucous membranes, which it moistens and protects.

MUMMERY
A term originally used to describe a kind of play in 17th century Europe, in which masked, costumed players performed stories which always ended happily regardless of the preceding events in the play. Often the happy ending was brought about by attributing supernatural skills to some character, e.g., a doctor might restore to life a character who had been killed. In the 18th and 19th centuries, the term became a euphemism for hypocrisy, especially for those who professed to cure through supernatural means, e.g., the "royal touch."

MUSH
Also hasty pudding.

MUST
The juice freshly pressed from grapes.

MUSTARD PLASTER
A plaster made of mustard or a mixture of mustard and flour to which enough water was added to produce a paste.
And powdered black mustard mixed with a solution of rubber.

MUTTERKORN
A remedy containing a fungus found on grain (usually rye). Used by midwives in Europe in the 19th century to promote contractions of the uterus.

MUTTERKRAUT
Also feverfew.

MYALISM
An ancient African religion wherein all illnesses were believed to be caused by the supernatural. Sorcerers were blamed for taking a sick person's soul and hiding it, thereby causing the illness. A sacrifice would be made along with chanting and dancing into a trance-like state until the soul returned to the body of the sick person.
And, beginning in colonial times, an anti-white secret society that existed until the early 1900s.

NARCOTIC
A drug that promotes sleep, relieves pain and produces unconsciousness. Until the early 20th century, this was a generic term that included alcohol as well as opium preparations.

NATES
Also backseat, buttocks, rump. The fleshy part of the body posterior to the hip joints.

NATUROPATHY
A drugless therapeutic system using only such physical forces as air, water, heat, light, diet, massage, etc. to ameliorate or cure diseases.

NAVAJO SINGERS
Navajo Native Americans believed that a family member could be cured of an illness by hosting a "sing." They gathered hundreds of Navajos to share the blessing of the chant.

NEAPOLITAN DISEASE
Also syphilis.

NECROSIS
Also sphacelus.

NERVINE
A remedy acting on the nervous system.

NERVOSITY
Excessive nervousness.

NERVOUS FEVER
Also typhus.

NETTLE RASH
Also hives.

NEURALGIA
Severe, throbbing, and episodic pain along a nerve tract. Different types were classified according to the part of the body affected, e.g., "sciatica" was the name for pain felt along the sciatic nerve tract, which runs from the back of a thigh and down the inner part of that leg. In the 19th century, they were also classified according to causes, e.g., malaria, syphilis, alcoholism, and hysteria.

NEUROSIS
A disorder of the nerves characterized by a loss of function in a part of the body without evidence of disturbance of the organ or system responsible for that function.
And, in psychiatry, a minor disorder of the mind.

NIGHTINGALE, FLORENCE

An Englishwoman who introduced the concept of sanitation as necessary to reduce mortality in the care of the sick and wounded. She demonstrated its effectiveness in the British military health care system in the mid-1800s.

NIGHTMARE

Also incubus.

NIT

The egg or larvae of a louse, usually attached to a hair.

NITER [NITRE]

Also saltpeter. A chemical compound found naturally in soil. It was largely produced in India, where soil was filtered to obtain the salt. Niter was also produced artificially by mixing animal and vegetable remains with ashes, lime, and loose soil. The whole mix would be turned over at intervals for 2 to 3 years. Used to treat fevers and as an antiseptic. The inhalation of fumes produced by burning niter paper was used to treat asthma.

NITER PAPER

Absorbent paper dipped in a solution of niter and dried.

NITROUS OXIDE

Also laughing gas.

NOCTURNAL ASTHMA

Also incubus.

NOMA

An inflammation of the mouth of children recovering from an eruptive disease. Characterized by the formation of a rapidly spreading gangrenous ulcer on the mucous membrane, it was usually fatal.

NOSTRUM

Also patent medicine.

NOTE BLINDNESS

A visual impairment in which the eye can no longer recognize or distinguish between written musical notes.

NOXA
That which is the cause of a disease such as a microbe.

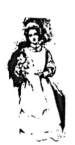

NURSEMAID
Also child-nurse.

NURSE'S CONTRACTURE
A condition occurring in nursing mothers characterized by painful spasms of the extremities, especially the arms. In the late 19th century it was believed to be caused by some unknown poison in the system of the mother. In the early 1900s it was found to be caused by a calcium deficit.

NUTGALL
Also galla.

NUX VOMICA
Also Quaker button.

OAK APPLE
Also galla.

OBEAH [OBIA]
An African American man or woman who practiced white magic to protect others from black magic. The obeah called up the spirits of the dead and prepared objects that were meant to kill an enemy, cure an illness, or win someone's love.

OBSTETRICS
Also tocology.

OCHLESIS
Any disease caused by overcrowding.

ODONTALGIA
Also toothache.

OIL OF WHELPES
A remedy for gunshot wounds concocted of newborn puppies, worms, and turpentine in the 16th century.

ONION
An herb used as a home remedy. It was believed to be helpful as a cough medicine and as a poultice.

OPIUM
The juice of the poppy used by the "regulars" during the second half of the 19th century as a remedy to relieve pain. Opium itself or its most popular derivative, morphine, was used. Many patent medicines contained opium. Addiction to both opium and morphine became a serious health problem as the 19th century ended.

ORACLE BONES
The Chinese art of healing was first found inscribed on bones dating back to the 14th century B.C. They were replaced with bamboo strips, then pieces of fabric until the creation of paper in the 1st century B.C.

ORDURE
Also feces.

ORIENTAL PLAGUE
Also black death.

OSTEOPATHY
A system of medical practice founded in 1874 by Dr. Andrew Taylor Still. He believed that diseases were caused by spinal injuries that interfered with the normal movements of the joints. Early osteopaths treated all diseases using only spinal manipulation. The spine was felt for variations from the normal position; any variations were then corrected by the hand of the physician moving the spine into proper alignment. The correction was believed to allow for a better blood supply and free flow of the "life force." Later osteopaths recognized the body as a neurally integrated whole, and they supplemented manipulation with massage, medicine, and surgery.

OUTHOUSE
Also privy.

OVERLYING
Accidental smothering of an infant due to the practice of the mother or nurse sleeping with the child. An 18th and 19th century term.

OXBILE
Also oxgall. Fresh bile from an ox was used as a remedy to stimulate the secretory activity of the liver and as a tonic and laxative.

OXGALL
Also oxbile.

OXYMEL
A syrup of honey and vinegar used as a vehicle for medicine.

OZENA
A chronic disease of the nose characterized by a foul smelling discharge and caused by inflammation of the nasal mucous membrane, syphilitic ulcerations, or dental decay.

PAGENSTECKER'S OINTMENT
A patent remedy containing mercury. Used by the "regulars" to treat eye inflammations.

PAIN IN THE SIDE
Pulmonary tuberculosis and pneumonia as identified in the 16th and 17th centuries.

PAINTER'S COLIC
Also lead colic, saturnine colic. A chronic condition caused by lead poisoning and characterized by severe abdominal pain, a hard shrunken abdomen, anemia, and muscle atrophy. Found in those

exposed to lead in industry, cosmetics, or from chewing lead toys or other objects covered with lead paint.

PALATINE FEVER
Also typhus.

PALMISTRY
Also chiromancy.

PALSY
Also paralysis.

PALUDISM
Also malaria.

PANDEMIC
A very widespread epidemic.

PAP
Infant food of soft consistency often made by mixing bread crumbs with cow's milk or water. Sometimes the food was pre-chewed by the mother or nurse before feeding it to the infant.
And nipple or teat.

PAPER FOODS
A term used in the early 1900s for foods that were lighter, especially vegetables, such as lettuce and celery.

PARALYSIS
Also palsy. A loss of motion or sensation in a part of the body.

PARALYTIC DEMENTIA
Also paretic dementia.

PARESIS
A partial paralysis, as in an incomplete loss of movement following a stroke.

PARETIC DEMENTIA
Also general paresis, paralytic dementia, progressive paralysis of the insane. A condition believed to be caused by syphilis or a severe nervous strain. Characterized by change of character, delusions of

grandeur, seizures, loss of muscular movement, and eventual paralysis.

PARVULES
Sugar-coated pills produced on a large scale in the late 19th century.

PASSIVE IMMUNIZATION
Also immunization.

PATENT MEDICINE
Also nostrum, quack medicine, secret medicine. Remedies usually concocted and prescribed by "irregulars." They were touted to cure all kinds of aches and pains, and most contained some form of alcohol or opium. Patent medicine appeared at the beginning of the 18th century and is associated with the enactment of the patent law and the development of newspapers and other advertising media.

PATENTS
English Americans in colonial times bought patents issued by the king of England which allowed them to make and sell remedies in America. The formulas for the remedies were owned by the patent holder and could not be sold by anyone else. To be patented the remedy had to be original. No proof of efficacy or safety was required.

PECCANT
Unhealthy or disease-producing.

PECTORAL CONDITIONS
A generic term used to indicate illnesses affecting the lungs such as bronchitis, whooping cough, pleurisy, and pneumonia.

PEDDLER [PEDLAR]
A traveling hawker selling small articles and remedies.

PEDICULUS
Also louse.

PELLAGRA
Also Lombardy leprosy, mayidism. A condition characterized by gastrointestinal disturbances, skin lesions, sores in the mouth, and

nervous and mental disorders. Until the early 1900s it was believed to be caused by eating diseased corn; later it was found to be a nutritional deficiency disease.

PEMBERTON'S COCA-COLA

A patent headache remedy and pick-me-up. Originally, it contained coca and was advertised as the "ideal tonic" in 1885.

PENIS

Also pizel.

PENNSYLVANIA GERMAN MAGIC FORMULA

Pennsylvania Germans believed in certain rules to cure an illness: the name of the patient was used; the disease was spoken to directly; actions were repeated three times; and some object was used to transfer the disease outside of the body. The object was then burned away, taking the disease with it.

PENNSYLVANIA GERMAN SPECIFIC REMEDIAL BELIEFS

Remove a foreign substance from the eye by rubbing the opposite eye.

A goiter can be cured by rubbing it with the hand of a corpse.

Seeing a person that you have not seen for a long time cures sore eyes.

Tie a string around your finger if you are forgetful.

PEPO

Also pumpkin seed. The seed from the fruit of a plant native to tropical America. Shelled or unshelled, the seeds were bruised and stirred up in a syrup in preparation for oral administration as a vermifuge.

PERIODIC FEVER

Also malaria.

PERKINISM

Also tractoration.

PERLOID

Also capsule.

PERNICIOUS ANEMIA

A chronic, progressive condition usually occurring in middle life and characterized by a very marked drop in the number of red blood cells in the body. Symptoms include tiredness, weakness, and frequent small amounts of bleeding into the skin or from the mucous membranes. In the 19th century it was a fatal disease, but in the mid-1900s it was found to be a vitamin B_{12} deficiency.

PERNICIOUS FEVER

Also sinking chills.

PERNIO

Also chilblain.

PERTUSSIS

Also whooping cough.

PERUVIAN BARK

Also Jesuits' bark.

PESTILENCE

Also plague.

PESTS (THE)

A common name used to indicate typhus and typhoid.

PEYOTE

Also mescal button. The dried top of a cactus plant considered to be a narcotic drug. It has been used by Native Americans in their religious rites to produce hallucinogenic states. The "regulars" used it to treat hysteria, insanity, asthma, and rheumatism.

PHENOL

Also carbolic acid.

PHILTER [PHILTRE]

A drug, substance, or magic spell believed to stimulate love.
And any magic potion.

PHLEGM

Thick, stringy, mucus secreted in the throat and upper air-ways and brought up by coughing.

And a "humoral" substance believed by ancient physicians to come from the brain. See **GALEN** and **HIPPOCRATES**.

PHLEGMASIA
A severe inflammation.

PHLEGMATIC TEMPERAMENT
Also lymphatic temperament. A name for the disposition of one who is easy going, expressive of feelings, and tending toward laziness. See **GALEN**.

PHLOGOSIS
Also inflammation. Morbid changes in tissues caused by some irritant and characterized by redness, heat, pain and swelling. Usually accompanied by a discharge.

PHOSPHONECROSIS
Also phossy jaw.

PHOSPHORUS POISONING
Also phossy jaw.

PHOSSY JAW
Also phosphonecrosis, phos- phorus poisoning. A condition characterized by deterioration of bone, especially of the lower jaw due to excessive exposure to phosphorus. Often experienced by workers in match factories.

PHOTOTHERAPY
The treatment of disease, particularly skin diseases, by light rays.

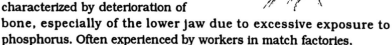

PHRENOLOGY
The study of the mind and character from configurations of the skull. It was based on the theory that each mental faculty was located in a fixed area of the brain and that the external configuration of the skull in-

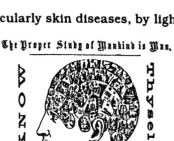

No. 308 Broadway, New York.
PHRENOLOGISTS and PUBLISHERS.

dicated the size and relative strength or predominance of each faculty.

PHRENZY
Also frenzy. A violent delirium that can occur in some cases of inflammation of the brain.

PHTHISIS
Also consumption, phthisis pulmonium, ptisic, tizzey, tyzie. Tuberculosis of the lung. A tubercular infection of the lungs characterized by the development of cavities that cause breathing difficulties along with a chronic cough. At first, the phlegm brought up by coughing contains purulent matter; later blood is expelled as well.

And a wasting of the body, local or general. A term commonly used during the 18th and 19th centuries but still found in current medical resources.

PHTHISIS PULMONIUM
Also phthisis.

PHYSICIAN
Also medicine man.

And also physitian. One who treats disease. In the 17th century many storekeepers, teachers, and ministers sidelined as physicians.

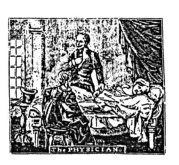

PHYSICIAN'S POCKET COMPANION
Also lancet.

PHYSICK [PHYSIC, PHYSICKE]
The science and administration of medicine.
And a cathartic.

PHYSITIAN
Also physician.

PIAN
Also yaws.

PICARDY SWEAT
Also sweating disease.

PIEBALD SKIN
Also vitiligo.

PIEN CH'UEH
A Chinese physician of antiquity, probably of Hippocrates time, called "the father of pulse" as he was the first one to diagnose illnesses by means of the pulse. Traditional Chinese doctors continued to place great importance on the pulse and a technique evolved that stressed gentle pressure on the pulse point to reveal the condition of the Yang organs and heavier pressure to reveal the condition of the Yin organs. Some Yang organs are the small intestine, gall bladder, and urinary bladder and some Yin organs are the heart, liver, and kidneys.

PILES
Blood-filled, venous swellings of the rectal mucous tissue, i.e., hemorrhoids.

PINKROOT
Also Carolina pink, Indian pink, star bloom, worm grass. An herbal remedy used by Native Americans as a vermifuge. It was adopted by the "regulars" who added calomel to the remedy.

PINTA [PINTO]
Also spotted sickness. A contagious tropical skin disease characterized by scaly pigmented patches of many colors mainly on the face and other exposed parts of the body. It was first noted in the 16th century by Cortes.

PINWORM
Also seatworm.

PIZEL [PIZZLE]
Also penis, yard. A sex organ of males.

PLAGUE
Also pestilence. Any disease of wide prevalence or of great mortality.
And **PLAGUE (THE)**. Also black death.

PLAGUE OF CIVILIZATION (THE)
Also dyspepsia. Disturbed digestion.

PLASTER
Also emplastrum. A solid, tenacious compound which can be spread on cloth or leather and which becomes adhesive when applied to the body. Plasters were used to keep the edges of wounds together, to protect raw body surfaces, and, when medicated, to redden or blister the skin for drug absorption.

PLEURA
The thin moist membranes covering the lungs and lining the cavity of the chest. Each lung is covered with its own pleural sac.

PLEURISY [PLEURITIS]
An inflammation of the pleura that may be classified as "dry" or "wet." The dry state is characterized by pain in the affected side, fever, and rubbing vibrations on the affected side. The dry state may become a chronic condition, or it may be followed by the wet state. The wet state is characterized by lessened pain and difficult breathing due to collection of fluid in the pleural cavity and on the pleural surface. The wet state also may become chronic. The major cause of pleurisy was tuberculosis, and sometimes it followed pneumonia.

PLUMPERS
Small ivory balls used to fill out the cheeks of those who had most of their teeth removed. Early 1800s.

PNEUMONIA
Also pneumonitis. An inflammation of the lung.
And an acute infectious disease characterized by fever, chest pain, cough, and blood-stained phlegm. Medical name is croupous or lobar pneumonia.

PNEUMONITIS
Also pneumonia.

PNEUMOTHERAPY
The practice of using air and gases to treat disease, such as the treatment of air sacs in the lung by continuous inhalation of oxygen.

POCULENT
Also potable. Describes a liquid, usually water, that is fit to drink as it will not cause illness.

POISON NUT
Also Quaker button.

POLISH DISEASE
Also syphilis.

POMADE
A medicated and/or perfumed ointment for the hair and scalp.

POMUM ADAMI
Also Adam's apple.

POORHOUSE
Also alms house.

POOR MAN'S GOUT
A condition similar to gout and believed to be due to hard work, exposure, ill food, and excessive drinking of malt liquor.

PORK WORM DISEASE
Also trichinosis. A disease caused by eating undercooked pork that contains trichina worms. Characterized early on by nausea, dizziness, fever, abdominal cramps, diarrhea--later by stiffness and painful swelling of the muscles.

PORRIGO
Any disease of the skin of the scalp and face characterized by the presence of dandruff-like scales. Includes ringworm and eczema.

PORTER
An alcoholic beverage having the qualities of beer and ale. It was believed to be so named because of its strong quality, which appealed to porters.

POSSET
A baby food made up of flour, sugar, and oil of sweet almonds or syrup of violets.

And hot milk curdled with wine, treacle, or acid.
And a mixture of beer and milk.

POTABLE
Also poculent.

POTASSIUM ARSENITE SOLUTION
Also Fowler's solution.

POTION [POTIO]
A large dose of liquid medicine or a liquid medicine taken in one swallow.

POUCH
Also medicine bag.

POULTICE
Also cataplasm.

POULTICING
Also fomentation.

POVERTY OF THE BLOOD
Also anemia.

POWDER OF SYMPATHY
A method of treating wounds in the 17th century. Attributed to alchemists, it was believed that a wound could be healed by treating the instrument that caused it. Salves or powders were applied to weapons that caused gunshot wounds. Or, in other types of wounds, sulfuric acid was poured on the purulent discharge found on the dressing removed from the wound.

POWWOW
Also conjure.

POWWOWING
Also brauching. The Native American's use of charms, incantation, and magic in ceremonies to cure disease and obtain success in war.
And also brauching. A European American folk medicine ritual using charms and physical manipulations to heal man and animal.

For example, Pennsylvania Germans would pass a hand over a sick person while looking at the waxing moon and chanting magic words. The term "powwow," derived from the language of New England Native Americans, became part the English language in the early 1600s. Some believe that this folk practice is traceable to medieval witchcraft cults.

POX (THE)
Also syphilis.

PRAIRIE ITCH
Also the itch.

PRAIRIE WOMEN
Women brought to mental asylums for depression caused by years of living in isolation on the prairies of Kansas and Nebraska.

PREVENTIVE INOCULATION
Also inoculation.

PRICKLY ASH
Also toothache tree.

PRIEST
Also medicine man.
And one who provides for the spiritual needs of a community.

PRISON FEVER
Also typhus.

PRIVY
Also backhouse, earth closet, outhouse. A small room away from the house where body wastes could be released.

PROGRESSIVE PARALYSIS OF THE INSANE
Also paretic dementia.

PROMINENTIA LARYNGEA
Also Adam's apple

PROPRIETARIES
Secret, patented, or trademarked, ready-made remedies.

PSORIASIS

A chronic inflammatory condition of the skin characterized by reddish patches covered with silvery scales. Itching does not usually occur. The cause remains unknown. In the 19th century, it was believed to be influenced by heredity, gout, rheumatism, dyspepsia, and lack of sunshine. Treatment included alteratives, cold baths, and ointment such as Alyon's.

PSYCHIATRIST

Also alienist.

PTISAN

Also tisane.

PTISIC

Also phthisis.

PUBLIC DRINKING CUP

A cup available to the public for drinking. One cup was used for drinking by all in public places, such as theaters, parks, and trains. The cup was usually attached to the water container. This practice continued in the United States until the early 20th century.

PUERPERAL FEVER

Also childbed fever. An acute, febrile disease due to a septic infection occurring in women after childbirth. It was believed to be a form of scarlet fever during the 19th century.

PUFFBALL

A fungus used as a by Native Americans and European Americans to control bleeding and relieve pain.

PUFFER

Also drummer.

PUFFERY

Also buncombe.

PUKE

A remedy that induces vomiting.
And a substance that is vomited.
And to vomit.

PUKEWEED

Also gagroot, Indian tobacco, lobelia, vomit root, vomitwort. An herb used in colonial times by Native Americans and European Americans for emetic and cathartic purposes. The leaves were frequently used as a substitute for tobacco or mixed with it. It was part of a patent remedy mixture for the cure of consumption and noted by the sellers to be an "Indian specific."

PUKING FEVER

Also milk sickness.

PULEX

Also jigger.

PULLIKIN

An instrument used by the country doctor to pull teeth in the 19th century.

PUMPKIN SEED

Also pepo.

PURGE

A strong cathartic.

And a purgative remedy or dose.

And to relieve of fecal matter by ingestion of a remedy, by clyster, or by treatment of the skin.

And **UPWARD PURGE**. Also vomitory.

PURULENT

Also suppurative. The condition of tissue containing or forming pus.

PUS

Also quitter. A liquid product of inflammation containing body fluids and debris from body cells. It usually has a yellow-white appearance, and it may or may not contain disease-causing microorganisms.

PUTREFACTION

The decomposition of organic matter into less complex substances. A decaying or rotting process.

PUTRID FEVER
   Also typhus.

PUTRID SORE THROAT
   Also gangrenous pharyngitis. An inflammation of the mucous membrane and underlying tissue of the throat that has progressed to the state where the tissue is dead. Characterized by pain, swelling, fever, and a foul smelling discharge from the mouth.

PYEMIA
   Also blood poisoning, septicemia. The presence of pus in the blood. Usually a fatal condition.

PYRETOTHERAPY
   Also fever therapy.

PYREXIA
   Also fever.

QUACK
   Also charlatan, codswallop, empiric. An individual who practiced medicine without the required skills. A term often used by the "regulars" about the "irregulars."

Quack Doctor

QUACK MEDICINE
   Also patent medicine.

QUAKER BUTTON
   Also nux vomica, poison nut, strychnine. A plant used in small doses as an herbal remedy and a bitter tonic for digestive prob-

lems, respiratory diseases, infectious diseases, and severe constipation.

QUARTAN FEVER

A form of intermittent fever where there is recurrence of the fever every fourth day.

QUARTERN

A generic measure used to indicate some parameter of the number four, e.g., a fourth of a peck or a four pound loaf of bread.

And also gill. A quarter of a pint.

QUASSIA

Also bitter ash, bitterwood. A remedy that was a simple bitter made from an infusion of the wood of the quassia tree, a tree of tropical America. It was used for stomach problems and as a clyster for destruction of seat-worms. A practical means of providing the remedy was to fashion a cup of the wood and allow water to stand in it overnight, refilling as needed. The name was taken from the African American man who first used the remedy in the early 1700s.

QUICKSILVER

Also mercury.

QUILLED BABY

A baby born of a mother who was treated with snuff blown into her nose with a goose quill during labor. The subsequent sneezing was intended to facilitate delivery.

QUINSY

A disease of the tonsils and mucous membranes of the throat characterized by inflammation and pus production around the tonsils.

QUITTER

Also pus.

QUOTIDIAN FEVER

A form of intermittent fever where there is recurrence of fever every day.

RABIES

Also hydrophobia, lyssa, St. Hubert's disease. An acute, infectious disease transmitted to man by the bite of animals infected with the disease. Characterized by paralysis of the muscles of respiration and swallowing, madness, and other symptoms of nervous origin. Until the latter half of the 19th century, it was usually fatal. There are records of this disease from antiquity.

RACHITIS

Also rickets.
And inflammation of the spine.

RAG AND BOTTLE

The first method of inhalation anesthesia. An anesthetic, such as ether, in liquid form was turned into a vapor by pouring it from a bottle onto a cloth.

RAGGED CUP

Also Indian gum.

RED ANT TREATMENT

A Mexican Native American remedy of red ants taken internally as an infusion or swallowed whole. For dysentery the red ants were externally applied to the abdomen. The entire body of the patient was covered by live red ants to treat rheumatism. In the early 19th century formic acid was found to be the active principle in the body of the ant.

RED CLOTH TREATMENT

In colonial times a red cloth was wrapped around a smallpox patient in the belief that it would prevent scarring.

RED GUM

Also gum rash, strophulus, tooth rash. A fine rash found on infants' skin at time of teething.

RED LIGHT TREATMENT
A form of phototherapy. A red glass or a thick red cloth was used to filter the light in the room of a smallpox patient in the belief that then the eruptions of smallpox would not become pus laden and form scars.

REFRIGERANT
A remedy that relieves fever and/or thirst, such as cool acidic drinks and evaporating lotions.

REGULARS
Properly qualified physicians conforming to the mainstream of medical practice as established in the first half of the 19th century. They were graduates of medical schools, and clinical practice and laboratory training were added during the second half of the 19th century.

REIN [REN]
Also kidney.

RELAPSING FEVER
Also famine fever.

REMEDIAL MASSAGE
Also Chinese remedial massage.

REMEDY
Anything that cures, treats, or prevents disease.

REMITTENT FEVER
Also malaria.
And a fever in which the temperature drops slightly but not back to normal in the periods between two pronounced episodes of high fever and/or chills.

REVULSION
A treatment for disease in which sudden withdrawal of blood was believed to divert the disease from one part of the body to another. One form of revulsion was blood-letting on the opposite side of the body from the disease; another was using counter-irritants on the skin.

RHEUMA [RHEUM]
Any watery or catarrhal discharge from the body.
And rhubarb.

RHEUMATISM OF THE WOMB
A condition of late pregnancy characterized by pain in the uterus. The treatment prescribed was the wearing of flannel drawers.

RICKETS
Also doubling of the joints, rachitis. A disease of infancy and childhood in which the normal process of bone development is disturbed. Characterized by bending and distortion of the bones, pain in the muscles, sweating of the head, and degeneration of the liver and spleen. In the mid-1900s it was found to be a deficiency disease.

RINGWORM
Also tinea. A generic term applied to a class of contagious skin diseases caused by fungi. Any part of the body can be affected. The specific characteristics vary according to location but generally include red, ringed patches of skin eruptions, itching, pain, and scaling.

RITUAL BATHING
A ceremonial practice of the Pacific Northwest Native Americans. They believed that it was a way of attaining special power for important tasks, including curing the sick. The seeker of the power abstained from normal activities of life and, during the waxing of the moon, bathed in icy water, chanting prayers while whipping the body with branches.

ROB
A jelly, confection, or thick syrup, especially of mulberries, used at times as a vehicle for medicines.

ROCKY MOUNTAIN TEA
A patent medicine, this remedy was an infusion of sage. Used for fevers when taken hot and as a tonic when taken cold.

ROENTGEN
Also x-ray.

ROETHELN
Also German measles.

ROOT DOCTOR
A folk healer in the South that used herbs and "rootworks" to treat disease. "Rootworks" were measures similar to powwowing considered essential to the treatment and taken to restore balance to the patient's life.

ROSE COLD
Also autumnal catarrh.

ROSIN WEED
Also Indian gum.

ROSY DROP
Also bottle nose.

ROWEL
Also seton.

ROYAL TOUCH
A ritual in which victims of scrofula sought cure. The kings of medieval England and France were believed to have special healing powers in their hands. Therefore, the king's touch or drinking the water in which he had washed his hands was considered a remedy for scrofula. Successors to these kings claimed such powers through the 18th century.

RUBELLA
Also German measles.

RUBEOLA
A generic term that includes measles and rubella.

RUMP
Also nates.

RUSH, BENJAMIN
A post-Revolutionary War physician. He believed and taught that there was only one disease and that a combination of vigorous purging and strenuous bloodletting would provide the cure.

SACK-'EM-UP-MEN

Also body snatchers, grave robbers. The procurers of corpses in the illicit trade in cadavers, which were in high demand for the purpose of dissection.

SACRED BARK

Also cascara sagrada.

SACRED DISEASE (THE)

Also epilepsy.

SAGE

Also salvia. An herb, native to southern Europe, whose dried leaves were used as a tonic, an astringent, and for fevers. Specifically, it was used as a gargle for inflammation of the throat.

ST. ANTHONY'S FIRE

Also ergotism, erysipelas, hospital gangrene. A generic name given for conditions characterized by inflammation and gangrenous manifestations on the skin. In the 19th century different causes of these signs of disease were found and other names were assigned as above.

ST. CATHERINE'S WHEEL

An amulet made in the image of the circular frame upon which St. Catherine suffered martyrdom. Some folk healers in the 16th and 17th centuries had the wheel tattooed on a part of their bodies to give credence to their ability to cure disease through supernatural means.

ST. GOTTHARD'S TUNNEL DISEASE

Also hookworm disease.

ST. HUBERT'S DISEASE

Also rabies.

ST. JOHN'S WORT
A plant used as an herbal remedy by voodoo conjurers and other folk healers to treat everything from dysentery to pulmonary ailments. It was best known for its magical powers to heal and was given the name "John de Conker" (Conqueror).

ST. ROCH'S DISEASE
Also buboes.

ST. SEMENT'S DISEASE
Also syphilis.

ST. VITUS' DANCE
Also chorea. A functional nervous disorder characterized by involuntary actions of the muscles.

SALIVATION
An excessive discharge of saliva from the mouth often associated with mercurial treatment.

SALTPETER [SALTPETRE]
Also niter.

SALT RHEUM
Eczema of the hands.

SALUTARY
Favorable to the preservation and restoration of health.

SALVIA
Also sage.

SANGUINE TEMPERAMENT
A name for the disposition of one who is energetic and hopeful with a quick but short-lived temper. See **GALEN**.

SAPO
Also soap.

SARSAPARILLA
A plant whose root was used to make a tea for treatment of syphilis, gout, rheumatism, tuberculosis, and fevers. It was believed

to be a blood purifier and was commonly taken as a spring tonic. A carbonated drink flavored with it was sold at soda fountains in the early 1900s.

SASSAFRAS TREE
Also ague tree, cinnamon wood, saxifrax. In the late 1600s it was promoted as a cure-all; Virginia colonists collected the bark and sent it to England. In traditional medicine, a tea made of the bark of the root was used as a remedy for blood purification, rheumatism, gout, arthritis, and skin problems. The inner part of the stems was used for eye poulticing and made into a drink for cases of dysentery and kidney disease. The root was popular as a tonic and became an ingredient in root beer. Native Americans made a tea from the root to treat fevers.

SATAN'S APPLE
Also European mandrake, man root. The root of this plant was used in ancient medicine to treat pain and melancholy and to promote fertility. The root's resemblance to the human form was the basis for a supernatural fear of the plant; it was believed that those who pulled the roots could die. Dogs were trained to pull the roots for the collectors of the plant.

SATURNINE COLIC
Also painter's colic.

SAXIFRAX
Also sassafras.

SCABIES
Also the itch.

SCALD-HEAD
Also scall. A condition of the scalp characterized by scaly and purulent skin eruptions.

SCALL
Also scald-head.

SCARFSKIN
Also epidermis, scurfskin. The outer layer of skin.

SCARIFICATION

The making of a set of small, superficial incisions or punctures in the skin with a mechanism that consisted of several lancets operated by a spring mechanism.

And the process of vigorously scraping the intact skin over a swelling.

SCARLATINA

Also scarlet fever, scarlet rash. An acute, contagious disease characterized by fever, sore throat, and rash. Kidney disease was a frequent complication. It was often confused with measles. The disease was first described in the latter half of the 17th century.

SCARLATINA RHEUMATICA

Also dengue.

SCARLET FEVER

Also scarlatina.

SCARLET RASH

Also scarlatina.

SCHIRRHOUS [SCIRRHOUS, SCIRRHUS]

A hardening of tissue, especially that preceding cancer.

SCHNAPPER

Also fleam.

SCHWEISSFREISEL

Also sweating disease.

SCHWITZGEGREIDER

Also sweat herbs. Pennsylvania German remedies for fevers that included chamomile, feverfew, and the mint family.

SCOLDING BRIDLE

Also branks.

SCOURGE OF NATIONS

Also cholera.

SCOURING

Also flux, lask. A severe diarrhea. The term was first used to indicate severe diarrhea in farm animals.

SCRIVENER'S PALSY

Also writer's cramp. An occupational disorder due to repeated use of the hand, as in writing.

SCROFULA

Also king's evil. A term first used to identify a constitutional condition usually found in the young and characterized by enlarged glands and the breakdown of bony tissue It was discovered to be a form of tuberculosis in the late 1800s. Some believed that it could be cured by a king's touch and the term "king's evil" became attached to this condition.

SCROTUM

Also cod. The sack containing the male glands that produce semen.

SCRUM POX

Also impetigo. A contagious disease of the skin characterized by inflammation and pustular eruptions, usually around the mouth and nose.

SCURFSKIN

Also scarfskin.

SCURVY

Also mouth badness. A condition that was found in those who had been deprived of proper food for a length of time. It was characterized by spongy gums, bleeding beneath the skin and mucous membranes, and foul breath. Prior to the 19th century, it was common among sailors and those who made long ocean trips. It was noted that those individuals eating fruits and/or juices of fruits did not get this condition, and a fruit ration became part of the diet of the sailor. Scurvy became known as a deficiency disease in the early 1900s.

SEA ONION

Also squill.

SEA THERAPY
A treatment that was based on the belief that healing could be achieved by sea baths, sea voyages, and/or seaside activities.

SEATWORM
Also pinworm. A small, parasitic, white worm that was found in the lower bowel and, occasionally, in the female genitals and bladder. Often found in the rectums of children, it caused severe itching.

SECRET DISEASE
Also venereal disease.

SECRET MEDICINE
Also patent medicine.

SEGENSFORMEN
A German ritual to cure disease by magic formulas and the laying on of hands. Similar to powwowing, it is believed to have been practiced since medieval times.

SELF-DOSAGE
Homemade remedies that were administered at home were the first line of prevention and therapy by which people sought to combat disease. Knowledge of these remedies was based on both the natural and magical/religious parts of folk medicine passed on through oral tradition.
And also domestic medicine.

SENECA SNAKEROOT
Also snakeroot.

SENILE ATROPHY
Also marasmus senilis.

SEPSIS
The poisoning of the body by the presence of disease-causing organisms and their products in the blood or tissues.

SEPTIC
Pertaining to or produced by putrefaction.

SEPTICEMIA
Also pyemia.

SEPTIC SORE THROAT
Also malignant sore throat.

SERPIGO
A generic term for any creeping skin eruption, such as ringworm or herpes zoster.

SETON
Also rowel. A twist of cloth or thread introduced into a wound to augment drainage.
And a thread introduced under the skin to cause blistering.

SHADOWGRAM
Also x-ray.

SHAMAN
Also medicine man. An Asian term given to the Native American medicine man by ethnologists to reflect a similar belief of both cultures, i.e., that the behavior of good and bad spirits can be controlled only by the individual assigned to this role.

SHAMPOOING
A form of massage in which the fingers are pressed and moved over the surface of the body. Used with malaxation to treat sterility in men in the early 19th century.

SHELL SHOCK
Also sinistrosis, war neurosis. A general term used to cover all serious mental and nervous conditions resulting from engagement in warfare during World War I.

SHINGLES
Also herpes zoster, zona. An acute, inflammatory condition of the skin and mucous membranes characterized by groups of small blister-like eruptions usually on one side of the body and associated with pain.

SHIP FEVER
Also typhus.

SHODDY FEVER

A disease believed to be caused by the inhalation of lint dust generated in factories that made wool fabric. Characterized by fever, headache, cough, and breathing difficulties.

SHOTGUN PRESCRIPTION

A remedy that contained numerous ingredients given with the hope that one or more might be effective.

SHOW GLOBES

Bottles of unusual shapes filled with colored liquids which have been used since the 17th century to attract customers into the apothecary shop or drug store.

SICK

Also courses.

SICK HEADACHE

Also migraine.

SICK-NURSE

In the 18th and early 19th centuries, a woman without formal training who cared for the sick.

And in the second half of the 19th century, a woman who after a year of training carried out her nursing duties under the supervision of a physician. Often this role would be combined with the duties of a nursemaid.

SICK STOMACH

Also milk sickness.

SIEGE

Also feces.

SILPHIUM

Also Indian gum.

SIMPLE BITTER

A disagreeable-tasting herbal remedy that affects only the stomach and intestine.

SIMPLES
Herbal remedies made up of a single herb.

SINGULTUS
Also hiccough.

SINISTROSIS
Also shell shock.

SINKING CHILLS
Also pernicious fever. A serious form of chills and fever which was usually fatal.

SIRRUP [SIRUP]
Also syrup. A concentrated, sticky solution of sugar, water, and other flavorings, often medicated.

SITZ BATH
Also hip bath.

SKIM MILK
Also fleet milk. Milk which has had its cream removed.

SLABBER [SLOBBER]
Also slaver.

SLAVER
Also drivel, slabber, slobber. The involuntary discharge of saliva from the mouth.
And saliva that has flowed out of the mouth.

SLEEPING SPONGE
A sea sponge saturated with mixed juices of sleep-producing plants. The fumes were inhaled by the patient before an operation. It was introduced in the 9th century and was the major anesthetic of the Middle Ages.

SLOUGH
Also sphacelus.

SLOWS (THE)
Also milk sickness.

SMALLPOX
Also variola.

SMOKE TREATMENT
Also Indian smoke treatment. A Native American remedy for respiratory and rheumatic illnesses. Cedar branches or sweet smelling herbs were heated or burned over live coals and inhaled by the patient.

SNAKEROOT
Also milkwort, mountain flax, seneca snakeroot. A plant whose roots were used as an herbal remedy. European Americans used it as an expectorant for breathing problems. The Seneca tribe of Native Americans applied it to snakebite wounds after cleaning out the venom.

SNOW COLD
Also autumnal catarrh.

SNUFFLES
Catarrh of the nasal passages. Commonly found in newborns of syphilitic mothers.

SOAK (A)
Also tippler.

SOAP
Also sapo. A compound of oils or fat with an alkali. Used as a cleansing and washing agent and as a remedy for various conditions. Usually given with rhubarb, it was used internally as a laxative, an antacid, and to prevent kidney stones. Externally, it was used to heal sores and cure the itch. Soap clysters were given for constipation. Pharmacists used it to make pills. These remedial uses continued through the first half of the 20th century.

SODA WATER
A remedy of carbonated water containing a medicinal ingredient, or artificial mineral water. Prescribed in the late 18th and early 19th centuries. Later it was used to create soft drinks, and soda fountains became popular.

SOFTENING OF THE BRAIN
Also encephalomalacia.

SOOT
A black, carbon substance condensed from smoke. Prescribed in tea as a tonic or to relieve spasms and, externally, for skin diseases and to control hemorrhages.

SOOT CANCER
A cancer of the scrotum frequently found in men employed as chimney sweeps.

SORCERY
Also black magic, witchcraft. The art which was supposed to make use of the power of evil spirits over others.

SOSTRUM
A fee for a physician's service.

SPANISH DISEASE
Also syphilis.

SPANISH FLY
Also cantharides.

SPANISH INFLUENZA
Also influenza.

SPANISH WINDLASS
Also garrote tourniquet. A form of tourniquet consisting of a handkerchief tied about a part of the body and twisted by means of a stick.

SPECIES
A mixture by the apothecary of coarsely cut or bruised parts of plants, trees, mosses and lichens, seeds and fruit to be made into a remedial tea.

SPELTER SHAKES
Also metal fume fever.

SPHACELUS

Also gangrene, necrosis, slough. A mass of dead, soft tissue in or separated from living tissue.

SPIDER CANCER

Also bottle nose.

SPIDER WEB

A remedy of Native Americans and European Americans until the early part of the 20th century. The cobweb spun by the spider was rolled into pill form and taken to reduce fevers or relieve spasms and as a sedative. Locally, it was used to stop bleeding in skin ulcers and after tooth extractions. It was also found to be useful as a moxa. The spiders themselves were used to treat malaria.

SPIRIT

The vital force or soul.
And any alcoholic solution obtained by distillation.

SPIRIT-RAPPING

The practice of knocking on wood to ward off evil. Oak was the only kind of wood considered effective for spirit-rapping.

SPIRITS [SPIRITUS]

An alcoholic beverage, stronger than wine, used by the pharmacist to prepare remedies.

SPIRITUS FRUMENTI

Also water of life.

SPIT CUPS

Personal containers used by individuals with tuberculosis of the lungs to catch materials brought up by coughing.

SPITTLE

A hospital for those afflicted with leprosy in 17th century England.

SPLEEN

Also lien, milt. A large, internal organ found on the upper left side of the abdominal cavity. Its function is believed to be to maintain a normal amount of healthy blood cells through the formation and storage of new cells and the destruction of old cells. It is not essential to life. In the 20th century, removal of the spleen did not cause death as was previously expected. The melancholic humor was believed to be found in the spleen. See **BLACK BILE**.

SPLENIC FEVER
Also anthrax.

SPOON MEAT
Liquid or semi-liquid food fed with a spoon.

SPOTTED FEVER
Also typhus.

SPOTTED SICKNESS
Also pinta.

SPRING WATER
Water from natural springs was used by Native Americans as a remedy for rheumatism, fever, backache, chest or stomach pains, and weak or sore eyes. Mineral water from springs found in North America and Europe was a popular remedy used by European Americans during the latter half of the 19th century for rheumatism, gout, and general well-being. They drank the water and bathed in it.

SPRUCE BEER
A remedy made by boiling the tops of spruce boughs in beer. Used to treat scurvy in the 18th century.

SPRUCE TEA
A remedy, similar to spruce beer, drunk by California gold-rushers of 1849 for scurvy.

SQUILL
Also sea onion. The bulb of a plant native to southern Europe and in the same family as onions and leeks. It had been used since ancient times to treat dropsy. In the 18th and 19th centuries, it was used mainly for respiratory conditions.

SQUILL SYRUP
Also hive syrup.

STAB-FREES
Also kugelfest.

STARBLIND
A condition in which an individual stares with eyes half closed, appears to be slow to understand, and blinks frequently.

STAR BLOOM
Also pinkroot.

STERNUTATORY POWDER
A remedy that is used to produce sneezing.

STICK-FREES
Also kugelfest.

STIFF NECK
Also wryneck.

STILLBORN
Also dead-born. An infant born lifeless.

STIMULANT
Also tonic.

STINKWEED
Also jimsonweed.

STITCH
A sharp pain in the side, at rib level, usually brought on by physical exertion, e.g., running or horseback riding. It ceases when the pace of the activity is reduced or stopped.

STITCHWORT [STICKWORT]
Also cocklebur. A plant native to Europe and North America. The entire plant was used to prepare remedies, e.g. alteratives and gargles. It was used specifically to treat a stitch. Native Americans used the root for fevers.

STOMACH
Also maw.

STONES
Also testes. Male glands found inside of the scrotum.

STOOL
Also feces.
And to empty the bowel of feces.

STOOLING
Continuous involuntary loss of feces from the anus.

STRANGURY
Slow and painful urination. The urine passes drop by drop due to spasms in the urinary passage and the bladder.

STRAWBERRY TONGUE
The red and swollen tongue found in individuals with scarlatina.

STREWING HERBS
Aromatic herbs, e.g., rosemary and lavender, that were scattered in areas where groups of people gathered. In the English Hall of Justice it was believed that the herbs would not only freshen the air but would also arrest the spread of the disease called "gaol fever." It was customary to present a bouquet of those herbs to the judge who presided at the proceedings in the Hall. Prior to the 20th century.

STROKE
Also apoplectic fit.

STROPHULUS
Also red gum.

STRUMA
Also bronchocele, goiter. A condition characterized by an enlargement of the thyroid gland causing a swelling in the front part of the neck.
And scrofula.

STRYCHNINE
Also Quaker button.

STUPE
A cloth dipped in hot water and then twisted to remove excess

water prior to application to the skin as a counterirritant. Turpentine was frequently mixed with the hot water.

SUBCUTANEOUS
Located under the skin.

SUCKING
A Native American treatment in cases of disease believed to be caused by a foreign presence in the body. Small cuts were made in the skin at the point beneath which the foreign object was thought to be. An animal's horn, a hollow bone or stick, or the mouth of the healer was used to suck the area and remove the object. This treatment is believed to have been used by many peoples in ancient and medieval times.

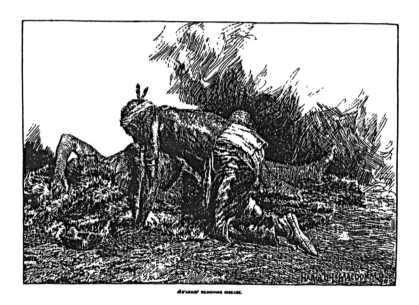

MEDICINE MAN REMOVING DISEASE.

SUDOR ANGLICUS
Also sweating disease.

SUETTE MILIAIRE
Also sweating disease.

SULFUR
Also brimstone.

SULFUR AND MOLASSES
A common home remedy for constipation in the 19th century.

SUMAC [SUMACH]
A tree whose leaves, bark, fruit, and root were used for remedial purposes in colonial America. Tea made from the bark was used for diarrhea. Tea made from the leaves and berries was used for urinary problems. Native Americans chewed the root to cure mouth sores. Some species of the tree are poisonous.

SUMMER COMPLAINT
Also cholera infantum.

SUN THERAPY
Also Chinese sun therapy.

SUPPURATIVE
Also purulent.

SURPRISE BATH
A treatment given to an insane or hysterical person prior to the 1900s. A sudden plunge into cold water.

SURGERY
Also chirurgery, chyrurgery. Medical treatment through procedures that require special instruments. In the Colonial period surgery included such things as amputations, repair of broken and dislocated bones, treatment of the skin, and cure of eye and ear conditions. Complex surgical procedures arose in the late 19th century with the increasingly widespread understanding of asepsis and the safe use of anesthesia.

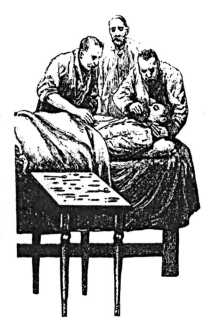

SURGEON
Also chirurgion, chyrurgion. A practitioner of surgery.

SWEAT BATH

Also Indian sweat bath. A common Native American way of socializing to maintain good relationships with others, of treating sickness, or of purifying the body before every important ritual. Believed to appease the spirits. The following is a general description: The bather was given a jar of water and a whip made of aromatic herbs; he entered a sweat lodge and stretched out or sat on a mat. Water was thrown on heated stones to produce the steam, and the bather whipped his body with the herbs until a heavy sweat was produced. The bath ended with a cold dip in a nearby stream or pond.

SWEAT DOCTOR

Also Indian sweat doctor. A special position in some Native American tribes. This person possessed some of the medicine man's power and had his own medicine song which was sung when the patient was treated in the sweat lodge. The song was the result of a vision or hallucination in which voices were heard.

SWEAT HERBS

Also schwitzgegreider.

SWEATING DISEASE

Also English sweat, miliaria, Picardy sweat, schweissfreisel, sudor anglicus, suette miliaire, sweating sickness. An epidemic disorder characterized by high fever, chills, and profuse perspiration lasting 2 to 24 hours and accompanied by fine skin eruptions. Death occurred rapidly after the symptoms appeared. It was prevalent in England, France, and Germany from the 16th to the 18th centuries. Some believe it to have been influenza.

SWEATING SICKNESS

Also sweating disease.

SWEAT LODGE

Also Indian sweat lodge. A small, low-domed hut made from willow sticks covered with animal skins. Entry required crawling through a low opening that was secured with a flap. Inside were stones which would be heated and have water thrown on them to produce steam.

SWEETMEAT
A confection usually made chiefly of sugar.

SWEET SPIRIT OF NITER [NITRE]
A volatile and inflammable liquid mixture of niter and alcohol. Used as a remedy for fevers, a diuretc, and an antispasmodic.

SWOON
Also faint, syncope attack. A sudden, temporary loss of consciousness, which can be partial or complete.

SYCOSIS
Also mentagra. A disease characterized by inflammation of the hair follicles, particularly of the beard. It was a chronic, pustular condition, most often found in a debilitated person. It was differentiated from a similar condition called barber's itch, which was known to be caused by a fungus.

SYMPATHETIC PRESCRIPTION FOR HERB GATHERING
Leaves plucked upward will be effective as an emetic, and leaves plucked downward as an enema.

SYNCOPE ATTACK
Also swoon.

SYNOVIAL FLUID
Also joint oil.

SYNTHETIC REMEDIES
As opposed to natural remedies, a generic term for complex remedies prepared from simpler compounds or elements by chemical means.

SYPHILIS
Also disease of Hispaniola, English disease, German disease, lues, mal Française, morbus gallicus, Neapolitan disease, Polish disease, the pox, St. Sement's disease, Spanish disease, Turkish disease. A chronic, infectious venereal disease named after a shepherd infected by the disease as documented in a poem written by Fracastorius (1530). Some believed that it had been spread by Spanish sailors returning from America in the late 1400s when it reached Italy and in a few years the whole of Europe. Others believe

that it was introduced to America by the Europeans that came to America in the late 1400s. In the 19th century it was noted to have three fairly definable stages: the primary stage, evidenced by an ulcer (chancre) and buboes; the secondary stage, evidenced by general enlargement of the lymph glands, eruptions on the skin, pustules on the mucous membranes and sore throat; and the third (tertiary) stage, evidenced by growths that undergo degeneration (gummata) in the organs or other tissues of the body. In the early 20th century it was noted that dementia and walking disturbances were part of the last stage of the disease in some patients, which suggested nervous system involvement.

SYRUP
Also sirrup.

TABES MESENTERICA
Tuberculosis found in the glands of the lining of the abdomen in children. Characterized by progressive wasting.

TABOO [TABU]
A sacred prohibition or restriction, resulting from convention or tradition, laid upon a person, place, day, name, or other object.

TABOO VIOLATION
A belief of the Native American that members of the tribe who hunted animals or gathered herbs must always sing the required songs or prayers, or offer gifts of tobacco to the spirits of the animals, plants, or objects. Failing to do so would offend the spirit and lead to illness or bad luck.

TAENIA [TENIA]
Also tapeworm. A parasitic, segmented worm that attaches its head to the intestine of a human or an animal. It can be transmitted to humans through the uncooked meat of an infested animal.

T'AI-CHI [T'AI CHI CHUAN]

Originally a Chinese martial art of fisticuffs for monks. In the 10th century it evolved into therapeutic exercises, the purpose of which was to obtain mastery over the body by means of both inward calm and physical exercises done in a slow, loose manner. Once mastery was achieved it would be possible to overcome any attack on one's health.

TANNIN

An acid substance found in the nutgalls on trees and in tea. It was used as an astringent for catarrh of mucous membranes and on skin diseases. Tanneries were so named because of their use of this substance in making leather from animal hides.

TAOISM

A Chinese philosophy and religion, originating in the 6th century B.C., that advocated simplicity and selflessness. Taoism views illness and health as phenomena that affect all persons equally. The Taoist hermit-physician meditated, treated peasants and royalty, and searched for new remedies. Other Taoist healers were involved with alchemy and magic.

TAOIST MAGICIAN

A Taoist alchemist practicing mainly in the court of the Chinese Emperor and seeking the "the elixir of life." Some believed mercury, especially blood-red cinnabar (the principle ore of mercury), to be the source of the magic remedy that could confer immortality. Cinnabar was also known as dragon's blood.

TAPEWORM

Also taenia, tenia.

TAR WATER

A remedy that was believed to be a cure-all and became, for some, an alternative to inoculation against smallpox. A cold infusion of tar water was produced by shaking one quart of water with one quart of tar (the resin obtained from evergreens) and allowing the tar to settle. When a glass was poured off and taken as a remedy, it was replaced with fresh water and shaken again for further use.

TARWEED
Also yerba santa.

TATTOOING
A form of picture writing that originated in ancient times and continues to the present day. It includes permanent marking of the body with coloring matter intro-

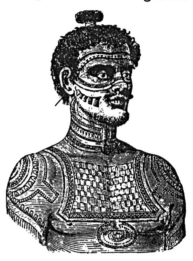

duced under the skin, scarification, and body painting. Native Americans used tattooing for the treatment and prevention of disease, to make the skin resistant to weapons, to scare the enemy, and to appease the spirits. It was originally developed among many primitive people as a means of protection from evil spirits. Early American sailors believed that a pig tattoo on one foot and a rooster tattoo on the other would prevent drowning. The crowing rooster was believed to drive away evil.

TEA [TEE]
A shrub native to China whose leaves are used in an infusion to produce a drink called "tea." Known since antiquity, it contains caffeine and tannin. Medici-

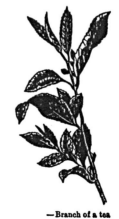

nally, it was given as a stimulant and to relieve headaches. It was applied to relieve eye inflammations and skin affections. North American colonists were very fond of this beverage. In the 19th and early 20th centuries some physicians and religious groups considered it, along with coffee, to be a habit-forming drug in the same category as alcohol and tobacco.

And an infusion of a medicinal plant.

—Branch of a tea plant.

TEETHING

Also cutting of the teeth. The eruption of a baby's milk teeth beginning about the seventh month of life. In the 18th, 19th, and early 20th centuries it was believed that teething was a serious problem of childhood as it caused cough, diarrhea, wasting, convulsions, and death. Treatments by the "regulars" included purging and scarification with a lance.

TENDERS

Women who were care takers of infants or sick persons in the 18th century.

TENDER TOES

A condition found in typhoid fever patients due to impaired circulation in the feet causing pain to such an extent that a tent was placed over the feet to protect them.

TENESMUS

Straining, especially ineffective efforts at stool or urination.

TERTIAN FEVER

An intermittent fever recurring every other day.

TESTES

Also stones.

TETANUS

Also lockjaw, trismus. An acute, infectious disease resulting from a puncture wound and characterized by painful, unremitting muscular contractions. Hippocrates recognized this disease.

TETOTUM ELECTICUM

A four-sided device used to select remedies to treat the sick. It had pasted on its sides the initials of various remedies. The tetotum would be twirled and when it came to rest the letter which came out on top indicated the remedy to be given.

TETTER

Also milk crust. A generic name for skin eruptions, particularly herpes, eczema, and psoriasis.

THE LONG LOST FRIEND
America's most popular folk medicine manual, which was written by John Hohman and published in Pennsylvania in 1819. Believed to have been the most popular conjuring book in this country.

THERAPEUTIC TRAVEL
A treatment for illnesses, especially consumption, consisting of a complete change of environment. After the Civil War, it was prescribed more for maintaining health.

THERAPY
The treatment of disease.

THERIACA
Also galene, Venice treacle. A compound originally containing more than 70 ingredients, including herbs, minerals, meat, honey, opium, and wine. It was believed to be an antidote against the poison of animals. It was first prescribed by Galen in the 2nd century and continued to be used through the 18th century.

THERIODIC
Malignant.

THEURGIST
Also medicine man.
And one who has access to supernatural means of controlling events.

THOMSONIANISM
A system of botanical medicine created by Samuel Thomson, an itinerant herb and root doctor, in the early 1800s. He promoted his system through his book on home-prepared medicine. Public support for his system was nationwide at that time.

THORN APPLE
Also jimsonweed.

THOROUGHWORT
Also boneset.

THROWING AWAY

A Quaker phrase for the behavior of Native Americans when they abandoned their old and sick to die due to the belief that the old and sick were possessed by evil spirits.

THUNDER BOX

Chinese container for excrement.

TICK

Also mite.

TINCTURES

Remedies made up of minerals, corals, rust, orange peels, red rose petals, aloes, etc. which were softened in alcohol, during the 16th and 17th centuries.

And remedies made up of vegetable and animal drugs macerated in alcohol, during the 18th and early 19th centuries.

And remedies made up of alcohol and medicine, beginning in the mid-19th century.

TINEA

Also ringworm.

TIPPLER

Also a soak. A bibulous person, that is, one who habitually drinks alcoholic beverages.

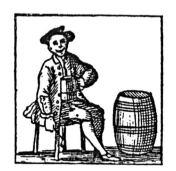

TIPPLING

Steady drinking of alcoholic beverages.

TISANE

Also ptisan. A medicinal drink prepared as a decoction from a variety of plants, e.g., aloe, chamomile, and barley.

TIZZEY

Also phthisis.

TOBACCO

The dried leaves of a plant containing nicotine. Native Americans believed that it would bring good and arrest evil in such matters as food, weather, and enemies. It was smoked in pipes to indicate hospitality and in ceremonial pipes during rituals to guard the welfare of the tribe. They mixed it with bearberry or sumac leaves as a remedy to treat phlegm. European Americans considered it to be a cure-all. Pennsylvania Germans chewed the plant to prevent and cure toothaches and blew the smoke into the ear to kill the insect that caused insanity. It was used world-wide as a sedative, being smoked, chewed, or snuffed.

TOCOLOGY [TOKOLOGY]
Also obstetrics. That part of medicine that deals with the care of women during pregnancy, labor and delivery, and the puerperium.

TOE ITCH
Also ground itch.

TOMATO
Also love apple. The berry of a plant that was believed to be poisonous until the 19th century. By the early 1900s it was known to be rich in vitamins. Physicians, at that time, considered it to be injurious in the diet of a gouty person.

TOMBSTONE HOOTCH
Also moonshine.

TONIC
Also bracer, stimulant. A 19th century remedy that was believed to give strength to the body as noted by changes in appetite, digestion, and color of skin. Before the Civil War arsenic was a favorite tonic. Quinine and strychnine became favored after the Civil War. Beverage alcohol became the most important tonic for children and adults during the second half of the 19th century. Homemade tonics consisted of whiskey or brandy with herbal tea.

TOOTHACHE
Also odontalgia. Pain in a tooth or the area around the tooth due to dental decay. Until the mid-1700s, it was believed to be due to the gnawing of a worm.

TOOTHACHE BUSH
Also toothache tree.

TOOTHACHE TREE

Also prickly ash, toothache bush. A remedy made from the bark of this tree was used by Native Americans for toothaches. Early settlers considered it a home remedy for toothache, colic, and rheumatism. African Americans in the South used it for toothaches and rheumatism.

TOOTH CARE

Also African American tooth care. In the 18th century, African Americans cleaned their teeth using an orange tree sprig that was bitten at one end until the fibers became brush-like. It sweetened the breath at the same time. Native Americans, too, used sprigs from plants or trees to clean their teeth.

TOOTH RASH

Also red gum.

TOOTH SPASM

Also infantile eclampsia.

TOPER'S NOSE

Also bottle nose.

TORMINA

Severe colic or griping intestinal pain.

TORPOR

Extreme sluggishness in ability to respond to stimuli.

TORREFIED

Dried with the aid of high heat, roasted, or scorched, as in the pharmaceutical preparation of some medicines.

TORTICOLLIS

Also wryneck.

TOWEL BATH

Also cold towel rub. A therapeutic bath in which the body was rubbed briskly with a wet hand towel using one quart of cold water. The towel was dipped into the water, squeezed out, and redipped as necessary to keep it slightly wet. The towel was placed on a part of the body, which was then rubbed. This process was repeated until arms, legs, chest, and back had been treated.

TRACHITIS [TRACHEITIS]
Also croup.
And inflammation of the windpipe (trachea).

TRACTORATION
Also perkinism. A form of metallotherapy. The treatment of disease by metal tractors. A tractor (two metal rods, formed of different metals, about three inches long and joined at one end to form a "V") was waved over the body. It was popular during the mid-1700s.

TRADITIONAL MEDICINE
The handing down of healing arts from generation to generation by oral communication.

TRANCE
Also animal magnetism.

TRANSPIRATION
The discharge of air, sweat, or vapor through the skin.
And material exhaled from the lungs.

TRANSPLANTATION
A process of healing in which the therapeutic substances applied to wounds would be removed and placed in a hole bored into an oak root. It was believed that the pain in the individual would cease if the material remained in the oak root.

TREACLE
Molasses.

TREMBLES (THE)
Also milk sickness.

TRENCH FOOT
A condition similar to frostbite, affecting the feet of soldiers, and due to prolonged exposure to the cold, wet trenches in World War I.

TRENCH MOUTH
Also mouth rot, Vincent's angina. An infectious disease of the

tonsils that extended to the floor of the mouth. Characterized by inflammation, ulceration, and painful swelling. It was found in soldiers that served in the trenches during World War I.

TRICHINOSIS
Also pork worm disease.

TRICKSTER
Also medicine man.
And a Native American term for a medicine man pretender who held no position of trust in the tribe.

TRILLIUM
Also birthroot.

TRISMUS
Also tetanus.

TRISMUS NEONATORUM
A form of lockjaw found in newborns due to infection introduced through the umbilical stump.

TROCHE
Also lozenge. A solid, flat tablet of medicine intended to dissolve in the mouth for its local effect on the mucous membranes of the mouth and throat.

TUBBING
A treatment for typhoid fever. The patient was placed up to the neck in a tub of warm water; the water temperature decreased over time, and then the patient was dried with a brisk skin rub.

TUBERCULOSIS
Also the great white scourge, white plague. An infectious disease characterized by small growths, called tubercles, that firmly embed themselves in tissues. The tubercles grow rapidly and die, thus destroying the surrounding tissues and resulting in cavities in the area of the body where they were located. Any part of the body could be affected and the symptoms would vary with the locality of the disease. Signs and symptoms common to all forms were loss of strength, anemia, fever, sweats, and emaciation. Person to person transmission of the disease was common as well as through

drinking contaminated cow's milk. In the late 1800s and early 1900s, it was considered the most widespread of human infections, and until the 1880s it was regarded as a constitutional disease.

TUBERCULOUS ARTHRITIS
Also white swelling.

TUMAH
A Jewish term for something which is ritually unclean, such as an unburied corpse or a death by suicide, which passes on its corruptness to all who are near.

TUMEFACTION
A swelling or tumor.
And sometimes used to indicate dropsy.

TUMOR
A morbid enlargement.
And a new growth that was not the result of inflammation.

TUNNEL ANEMIA
Also hookworm disease.

TURKISH BATH
A hot air bath in which the bather is moved from rooms of successively higher temperatures, from 95º to 160º Fahrenheit, then rubbed and splashed with cold water. Used to treat syphilis, chronic rheumatism, and general dropsy.

TURKISH BODY BAKE
Also body bake.

TURKISH DISEASE
Also syphilis.

TURPENTINE
Also turps. A remedy made from the resin of pitch pines. It had multiple uses. It was taken as a stimulant, to increase urinary output, to destroy intestinal worms, and, in large doses, as a laxative. Rectal injections were given for constipation. It was also believed to have a hemostatic effect. Used in ointments and lin-

iments to treat skin conditions. Turpentine stupes were used for abdominal distention. Chian turpentine from Asia, was sometimes used for the cure of cancer.

TURPS
Also turpentine.

TUSCARORA RICE
The first American-made patent remedy, introduced in 1711. It was made from corn and was advertised as a cure for tuberculosis.

TWILIGHT SLEEP
A state of clouded consciousness induced by the use of scopolamine (a cerebral sedative) and morphine (a narcotic), which were given during childbirth in the early to mid-1900s.

TYMPANITES
Also meteorism.

TYPHOID FEVER
Also abdominal typhus, enteric fever, filth disease. An acute, infectious disease characterized by fever, headache, abdominal tenderness, and diarrhea. Caused by bacteria carried in food and drinking water. Prior to the mid-1800s it was confused with typhus.

TYPHOID STATE
A condition of great weakness and stupor. It was characterized by a dry, brown tongue, teeth thick with oral debris, delirium, weak pulse, and loss of bowel and bladder control. It occurred in typhoid disease and other continued fevers.

TYPHUS
Also camp fever, gaol fever, jail fever, louse typhus, nervous fever, Palatine fever, prison fever, putrid fever, ship fever, spotted fever. An acute, contagious disease characterized by a fine rash, marked agitation and anxiety, and a high fever that lasted about two weeks. In the early 20th century it was found that the disease had two forms. The epidemic form was communicated through the bite of the body louse and the endemic form was communicated through the bite of the rat flea. One attack usually conferred immunity.

TYZIE
Also phthisis.

UBERTY
Also abundance.

UNCINARIASIS
Also hookworm disease.

UNFRUITFUL
Also barren.

UNWELL
Also courses.

UPWARD PURGE
Also vomitory. See **PURGE**.

URANIST
Also urning.

URBAN FEVER
A fever lasting about three weeks similar to typhoid except that specific symptoms were not present.

URNING
Also homosexual, uranist. Until the mid-1900s, a pervert; an individual exhibiting unnatural sexual preference for individuals of the same sex.
And, after the mid-1900s, an individual with sexual attraction toward those of the same sex.

URTICARIA
Also hives.

UTERINE ASTHMA

A female nervous disorder characterized by sudden, independent, upward movement of the uterus causing the compression of the liver and epigastric area (the upper middle abdominal area) to the degree that suffocation could occur. A form of hysteria first noted in the Middle Ages.

UTERUS

Also womb.

VACCINATION

An inoculation of cowpox that conferred immunity to smallpox in the early 19th century. It was found that inoculation with smallpox caused serious illness. As smallpox and cowpox were similar diseases and cowpox was a milder form, inoculation with cowpox was tried as a vaccine to prevent smallpox. It worked well to provide immunity to smallpox with a minimal reaction.

And, since the late 19th century, a general term to indicate inoculation with vaccine to prevent disease. See **IMMUNIZATION** and **INOCULATION**.

VACCINE DISEASE

Cowpox. See **VACCINATION**.

VALETUDINARIAN

Also invalid.

VANILLA

A tropical vine native to Mexico, whose pods (beans) are used to produce an extract used in perfume and as a flavoring agent for chocolate and ice cream. It has been used as a remedy for hysteria and low fevers. An infusion was prepared by mixing half an ounce of dry bean to one pint of water to be given in tablespoon doses.

VANISHING CREAM

Also greaseless ointment. A greaseless cold cream used in place of regular cold cream to cleanse the skin and remove blemishes. It was a patent cosmetic cream that was made up of stearic acid and glycerin, the ingredients of soap.

VAPOR

The condition of a liquid or solid when it becomes a gas by heating.

And a remedy to be administered in the form of a fume.

And **VAPORS (THE)**. An hysterical depression.

VARICELLA

Also chicken pox.

VARIOLA

Also continued fever, great leprosy, smallpox. An acute, highly infectious disease characterized by a sudden onset of high fever and diarrhea. On the third or fourth day another rise in fever occurs and skin eruptions begin, often leaving permanent scarring. It was noted in China and India around 200 B.C. and long has been regarded as native to India and Central Africa. In the 15th, 16th, 17th, and 18th centuries it was the cause of great mortality in many European countries. The wide decimation of the Native American from the 15th through the 19th centuries is believed to have been caused predominantly by smallpox.

VARIOLA CONFLUENCES

A severe form of variola in which the skin eruptions spread and run together.

VARIOLA MALIGNANT

Also variola nigra.

VARIOLA NIGRA

Also variola malignant. A severe and fatal form of variola in which there is hemorrhage into the eruptions, giving the skin a black appearance.

VARIOLATION

The inoculation of smallpox.

VENEREAL DISEASE

A contagious illness that is usually transmitted by sexual intercourse with an infected person.

And also secret disease. A generic term for gonorrhea, syphilis, and chancroid; they were grouped together until the 19th century.

VENEREAL SYPHILIS

Also syphilis.

VENICE TREACLE

Also theriaca.

VENTRICULUS

Also maw.

VERMIFUGE

A remedy that expels intestinal worms.

VERMIN

Originally meant worms, later became a generic term including other creatures believed to be harmful to humans such as lice, bedbugs, rats, mice, etc.

VERMINOUS

Infestation with worms or other vermin.

VERNIX

Also greasypaste.

VESICATORY

A remedy that produces a blister.

VESICULAR DERMATITS

Also eczema.

VICHY WATER

A mineral water remedy from a spring in Vichy, France. Used in rheumatism, gout, and disorders of the liver.

VINCENT'S ANGINA

Also mouth rot.

VINOUS INFUSION
A tea, made using wine as a diluent instead of water, to extract medicinal properties from a dry preparation of a remedy.

VIRUS
A contagium: the poison of an infectious disease, particularly one found in the secretions and tissues of a person or animal.

And, until the 1800s, lymph taken from vaccinated persons or persons recovering from smallpox, collected on the point of a transferring instrument, and applied to the skin of the person seeking immunity.

And, in the 20th century, an infectious agent, smaller than bacteria and generally not visible under ordinary microscopes. Some of the viral diseases of man are chicken pox, measles, smallpox, and the common cold.

VITAL AIR
Oxygen gas used as a treatment by inhalation for pulmonary conditions, severe anemias, suffocation, and opium poisoning.

VITAL RESISTANCE
The ability to endure hardship and to struggle for continued existence.

VITALS
A common term for the organs essential to life, such as the heart and lungs.

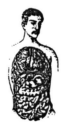

And a common term for measurement of vital signs.

VITAL SIGNS
Temperature, pulse, and respiration.

VITATIVENESS
Love of life and fear of death.

VITILIGO
Also piebald skin. An affection of the skin characterized by patchy disappearance of the natural pigment, leaving whitish areas.

It is more common in the tropics and in the Negro race, but the cause is unknown.

VOMITO NIGRO
   Also yellow fever.

VOMITORY
   Also emetic, upward purge. Any remedy that stimulates vomiting. European Americans and Native Americans believed that impurities in the body could be expelled from the mouth, and many of their remedies fell into the vomitory classification.

VOMITROOT
   Also pukeweed.

VOMITWORT
   Also pukeweed.

VOODOO [VODOUN, VUDU]
   An African cult that helped to provide for the needs of peasants by organizing large, extended families under the authority of a religious head man. There were many variants of voodoo, but generally the ceremonies take place outside, where chants and drums worked the participants into a state of trance. Purification by herbal water was part of the rite to protect them from any contact with death. The original form disappeared in the late 1800s and cult priests became simple healers. Africans taken into slavery brought voodoo with them to the West Indies in the 1600s. When Catholicism was introduced to them, they blended worship of the saints and God with the gods of Africa. In the 1700s, when voodoo came to the territory of the United States, its practice principally included witch doctors and black magic.

VOODOO DOCTOR
   Also hoodoo doctor. A folk healer who uses voodoo medicine.

VULNERARY
   A remedy that heals wounds.

WAMPUM

Native American beads made from shells. They were woven into belts or collars as symbols to sanctify transactions and were regarded as a very potent medicine. It was believed that failure to observe all the rules governing the transaction could bring illness or other misfortunes to the parties involved. Collars from beads made of glass or porcelain were brought from Europe by European Americans to bargain with Native Americans.

WANDERING DENTIST

An untrained person, usually a tinker (mender of kettles) with his own hand-made dental tools, who removed teeth. 19th and early 20th centuries.

WANG

The cheek.
And a molar.

WANGA

Black magic or witchcraft used by the African sorcerer in the form of charms and herbs to treat illness, to hypnotize, and to poison.

WARD'S ANODYNE PEARLS

A patent remedy made of beads worn on a necklace by teething infants.

WARD'S PASTE

A confection remedy of black pepper prescribed by the "regulars" for malarial fever in the early 19th century.

WAR NEUROSIS

Also shell shock.

WASHERWOMAN'S ITCH

Eczema on the hands of laundry workers. Caused by continual irritation from soapy water.

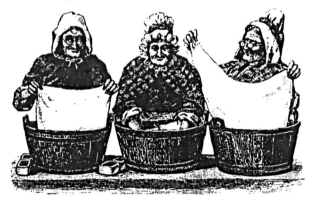

WASHLEATHER SKIN

A condition of the skin in which contact with certain metals, especially silver, mark it with a black line.

WASTING DISEASE

A chronic illness characterized by a loss of body weight and body strength, e.g., tuberculosis or cancer.

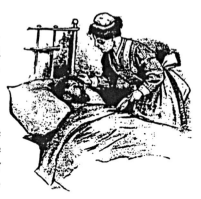

WATCHER

An assistant to a nurse. She replaced the nurse to allow the nurse respite time, usually while the patient was asleep. Mid-1800s.

WATCHMAKER'S CRAMP

An occupational neurosis occurring in watchmakers. Characterized by painful spasms in the muscles of the fingers.

WATER BRASH

Also brash. The belching up of small amounts of sour liquid.

WATER CURE

Also balneotherapy.

And a method of torture in which water was poured into the victim's mouth until choking occurred.

WATER HEAD
Also hydrocephalus.

WATER ITCH
Also ground itch.

WATER OF LIFE
Also spiritus frumenti. Whiskey obtained from the distillation of grain.

WATER ON THE BRAIN
Also hydrocephalus.

WATERY
Also hydronick.

WEASAND
A generic term for the opening from the back of the mouth into the body, that is, the gullet (esophagus) and the windpipe (trachea).

WEEPING SINEW
Also ganglion. A small swelling found on one or more of the tendons of the back of the wrist.

WET BRAIN
Also alcoholic cerebral edema. A condition found in all forms of alcoholism due to the retention of body fluids in the brain. Characterized by headache, nausea, and vomiting.

WET CUPPING
A form of bloodletting. It consisted of making small incisions on the surface of the skin and then increasing the flow of blood by suction.

WET NURSE
A woman who suckles (nurses) an infant in place of its mother.

WHELK

A generic term for an eruption on the face such as a pustule or tubercle.

WHISKEY [WHISKY]

A strong alcoholic drink made by the fermentation of malt. In diluted form it was used as a heart stimulant, digestive stimulant, beverage, and mild narcotic.

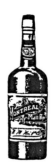

WHISKEY NOSE

Also bottle nose.

WHITE DRINK

A Native American name for a remedial tea made of holly leaves. Used as a stimulant and to induce vomiting. It was taken for various ceremonial purposes, such as purification through vomiting. It was called Indian Black Drink by the settlers in the late 1600s.

WHITE FLUX

Also cholera.

WHITE INDIAN DOCTORS

"Irregulars" who claimed to have learned their trade from Native Americans.

WHITE MAGIC

The art which was supposed to use supernatural and secret means to protect others from harm and to bring them good luck.

WHITE PLAGUE

Also tuberculosis.

WHITES (THE)

Also leucorrhea, leukorrhea. A whitish, purulent, vaginal discharge not containing blood.

WHITE SWELLING

Also tuberculous arthritis. A painful swelling of bone usually found in the joints. The skin remained white over the affected site due to an increase in the size of the bone. In the early 1900s it was discovered to be caused by a tubercular infection in the bone.

WHOOPING COUGH

Also hoopen cough, hooping cough, pertussis. An infectious, very contagious disease of children characterized by catarrhal inflammation of the air passages and peculiar spasms of cough with loud and deep inspiration. Complications included pneumonia and cerebral hemorrhage.

WILDCAT GREASE

A Native American remedy for wounds, aches, bruises, and rheumatism. The fat from the bobcat or lynx was rendered to a semiliquid state and applied to the body. Fats from many varieties of animals were common remedies for Native Americans.

WILD LEMON

Also May apple.

WILLOW BARK

A remedy used by Native Americans for fever. In the late 1700s it was used by the "regulars" as a substitute for cinchona to treat malaria. In the 19th century, chemists discovered the active substance in the bark which has come to be known by the trade name of "aspirin."

WINDINGO PSYCHOSIS

A cannibal syndrome found in some Native Americans of the Great Lakes area. Predominantly occurring in males, this psychosis was thought to be caused by possession by an evil spirit and a cold heart. Exhibited by a desire to eat family and friends, the resolution was execution performed by wife or other relative.

WINSLOW'S BABY SYRUP

A patent medicine in the late 1800s. A sleep-producing remedy for infants, the principle ingredient was morphine.

WITCHCRAFT

Also sorcery.

And also Indian witchcraft. Native Americans believed that witchcraft was practiced by those who were taken over by an evil influence making them different from other people. Those with the power of witchcraft were able to take other forms, and they traveled by night causing sickness and bringing bad luck to others. As with the European colonizers, often individuals identified as witches or sorcerers in Native American communities were put to death.

WITCH HAZEL WATER
Also hamamelis water.

WOMB
Also mother, uterus. The organ in which the unborn child is developed and kept until birth.
And belly or stomach.

WOOD ALCOHOL
Also moonshine.

WOOD SPIRIT
Also moonshine.

WOOLSORTER'S DISEASE
Also anthrax.

WORM GRASS
Also pinkroot.

WORT
A plant, herb, or vegetable.

WRITER'S CRAMP
Also scrivener's palsy.

WRYNECK
Also stiff neck, torticollis. A contracted state of the neck muscles, usually on one side, producing twisting of the neck and an unnatural position of the head.

WYMAN'S STRAPS
An arrangement of straps for holding a violent person in bed.

X-RAY

Also roentgen, shadowgram. The shadow picture made on a photographic film or plate by light rays possessing the power of penetrating objects impervious to other types of light. A late 19th century discovery of Dr. Wilhelm Konrad Roentgen of Germany.

YADIL

A patent remedy for influenza marketed in the United States during the influenza epidemic of 1918. It mainly contained garlic and water.

YARB

Also herb.

YARB AND ROOT DOCTOR

A practitioner who worked mostly with remedies obtained from the forest and the garden.

YARD

Also pizel.

YAWS

Also frambesia, pian. An infectious, tropical disease of the skin. Characterized by red eruptions commonly found on the face, toes, and genital organs. It resembled the skin manifestations of syphilis and was confused with that disease.

YEAST

A fungus used as a stimulant, or applied to the skin as a poultice for eruptions, or as a deodorant to gangrenous ulcers.

YELLOW BILE

Also choler. A light-colored "humoral" substance believed by ancient physicians to be from the liver. See **GALEN** and **HIPPOCRATES**.

YELLOW FEVER

Also American plague, vomito nigro, yellow jack. An acute, infectious disease of the tropical and subtropical regions of America characterized by degeneration of the liver and congestion of the mucous membranes in the stomach and intestines. Fever was present and hemorrhage of the mucous membranes was noted by the presence of black vomit. Death from this disease was frequent, the patient dying in the "typhoid state," often the result of kidney failure. It was unknown in America until the slave-trade was in full swing in the mid-1600s. It was the chief cause of death in the tropics during the 19th century.

YELLOW GUM

A sign of jaundice in children. The discoloration is noted in the mucous membranes covering the tissue that envelops the neck of the tooth and tooth supporting structures of the upper and lower jaw.

YELLOW JACK

Also yellow fever.

YELLOW ROOT

Also golden seal. A Native American herbal remedy believed to be a cure-all by Native Americans and European Americans. It has been referred to as the poor man's ginseng as it was believed to have similar powers and was readily available for collecting in the countryside.

YELLOW WAX

Also beeswax. The purified honeycomb of the bee. It was used to treat diarrhea and dysentery as it was believed that it healed the inflamed mucous membrane of the bowel. It has also been used in making candles, ointments, and pomades.

YERB

Also herb.

YERBA SANTA

Also bear's weed, consumptive's weed, gum bush, holy herb, mountain balm, tarweed. An herbal remedy believed to be a holy plant by the Spanish settlers in the 17th century. It was used to treat abundance of phlegm and other complications resulting from colds. In the 19th century it was believed to be a blood purifier and a cure for rheumatism and tuberculosis. Native Americans chewed or smoked the leaves as a cure for asthma.

YIN AND YANG

A doctrine of the art of healing from Chinese antiquity. It is believed that there is a constant struggle between opposing forces and that good or bad health is determined by the fluctuations of the conflicting forces of Yin and Yang. Yin includes negative, cold, dark, and female features reflecting passive moon energy; Yang includes positive, warm, light, and male features reflecting sun energy. Harmony between Yin and Yang results in good health; energy displaced in any way is revealed in poor health.

ZEA

Also corn silk.

ZEIST

A person who believes that pellagra is caused by eating poisonous corn.

ZIECKENTROOSTER

A person, usually a schoolmaster, assigned to treat the sick in the absence of a physician in 17th century Dutch colonies.

ZINC FUME FEVER

Also metal fume fever.

ZONA

Also shingles.

ZWISCHENTRAGER

An intermediate agent used in the magic ritual of German folk medicine to transfer a disease or condition away from the afflicted person. A common example of "Zwischentrager" was removal of warts with an agent such as salt or a raw potato which was rubbed on the warts and then disposed of to be picked up by some unknowing person or animal who would then get the warts. A form of folk magic.

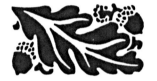

References

____. 1995. *Academic American Encyclopedia*. Vol. 14. Danbury, CT: Grolier, Inc.

Ackerknecht, E. H. 1955. *A Short History of Medicine*. New York: The Ronald Press Co.

Aikman, L. 1977. *Nature's Healing Arts*. Washington, D.C.: National Geographic Society Special Publications Division.

____. 1944. *The Album of American History in Colonial America*. New York: Charles Scribner's Sons.

Andrews, C. M. 1919. *Colonial Folkways*. New Haven: Yale University Press.

Ashburn, P. M. 1980. *The Ranks of Death*. Philadelphia: Porcupine Press.

Baker, J. T. 1907. *Correct English--How To Use It*. Baltimore, Maryland: The H. M. Rowe Co.

Bartholow, R. 1887. *Materia Medica and Therapeutics*. New York: D. Appleton & Co.

Bastide, R. 1971. *African Civilisations in the New World*. New York: Harper & Rowe Publishers.

Battey, T. C. 1875. *The Life and Adventures of a Quaker Among the Indians*. Williamstown, MA: Corner House Publishers.

Bettmann, O. L. 1974. *The Good Old Days--They Were Terrible*. New York: Random House Publishing Co.

Billard, J. B. 1974. *The World of the American Indian*. Washington, DC: National Geographic Society.

Billings, Frank, ed. 1915. *Forchheimer's Therapeusts of Internal Disease*. Vol. 2. New York: D. Appleton & Co.

Blair, E. H., ed. 1911. *The Indian Tribes of the Upper Mississippi Valley and Great Lakes Region*. Vol. 1. Cleveland: The Arthur H. Clark Co.

Blochman, L. G. 1958. *Doctor Squibb*. New York: Simon & Schuster Publishing Co.

Burt, A. L. 1882. *The National Standard Dictionary*. New York: A.L. Burt, Publisher.

Burton, R. 1620. *Anatomy of Melancholy*. Edited by F. Dell and P. Jordan. 1951. New York: Tudor Publishing Co.

Carson, G. 1961. *One For a Man, Two For a Horse*. New York: Bramhall House.

Cassedy, J. H. 1986. *Medicine and American Growth: 1800-1860*. Madison, WI: The University of Wisconsin Press.

Castiglione, A. 1947. *A History of Medicine*. New York: Alfred A. Knopf Publishing Co.

Clapesattle, H. 1943. *The Doctors' Mayo*. Garden City, NY: Garden City Publishing Co.

Cohen, A. A., and P. Mendes-Flohr, eds. 1972. *Contemporary Jewish Religious Thought*. New York: The Free Press.

Corlett, W. T. 1935. *The Medicine Man of the American Indian and His Cultural Background*. Springfield, IL: Charles C. Thomas Publishing Co.

Courlander, H. 1976. *A Treasury of Afro-American Folklore*. New York: Crown Publishing, Inc.

Cunningham, A., and R. French, eds. 1990. *The Medical Enlightenment of the 18th Century*. Cambridge, New York: Cambridge University Press.

Cutter, C. 1862. *Treatise on Anatomy, Physiology and Hygiene.* New York: Clark, Austin, Maynard & Co.

Davenport, F. M. 1905. *Primitive Traits in Religious Revivals.* New York: Macmillan Publishing Co., Inc.

Davenport, H. W. 1987. *Doctor Dock--Teaching and Learning Medicine at the Turn of the Century.* New Brunswick & London: Rutgers University Press.

Devens, C. 1992. *Countering Colonization.* Berkeley: University of California Press.

Donahue, M. P. 1985. *Nursing, the Finest Art.* St. Louis: The C. V. Mosby Co.

Dorland, W. A. N. 1944. *The American Illustrated Medical Dictionary.* Philadelphia: W.B. Saunders Co.

Dorson, R. M. 1959. *American Folklore.* Chicago: University of Chicago Press.

Eddy, M. B. 1875. *Science and Health with Key to the Scriptures.* Norwood, MA: The Plimpton Press.

____. 1892. *The Encyclopedia Britannica.* Volumes 6, 16, and 17. Chicago: R. S. Peale Co.

____. 1974. *The Encyclopedia of Magic and Superstition.* New York: Crown Publishers.

Ernest, R. 1991. *Weakness Is a Crime.* New York: Syracuse University Press.

Evans, N., P. T. Magan, and G. Thomason, eds. 1923. *The Home Physician.* Mt. View, California: Pacific Press Publishing Assoc.

Fantus, B. 1930. *General Technic of Medication.* Chicago: American Medical Assoc.

Fogel, E. M. 1915. *Beliefs and Superstitions of the Pennsylvania Germans.* Number 18. Philadelphia: American Germanica Press.

Gilbert, R. J. 1986. *Caffeine, the Most Popular Stimulant.* New York: Chelsea House Publishers.

Gilbert, S. 1989. *Medical Fakes and Frauds.* New York: Chelsea House Publishers.

Gottschall, S. 1973. *The Emergence of Christian Science in American Religious Life.* Berkeley: The University of California Press.

Gould, G. M. 1906. *The Practitioner's Medical Dictionary.* Philadelphia: P. Blakiston's Sons & Co.

Guide, R. E. 1989. *The Encyclopedia of Witches and Witchcraft.* New York: Facts on File, Inc.

Haggard, H. W. 1933. *Mystery, Magic, and Medicine.* Garden City, NY: Doubleday, Doran & Co., Inc.

Haller, J. S., Jr. 1981. *American Medicine in Transition: 1840-1910.* Urbana, Chicago, London: University of Illinois Press.

Hand, W. D. 1980. *Magical Medicine.* Berkeley: University of California Press.

Handlin, O. 1949. *This Was America.* Cambridge, MA: Harvard University Press.

Harpole, J. 1937. *Leaves From a Surgeon's Case-Book.* New York: The New Home Library.

Hawke, D. F. 1971. *Benjamin Rush.* Indianapolis & New York: The Bobbs-Merrill Co., Inc.

Heiser, V. 1936. *An American Doctor's Odyssey.* New York: W. W. Norton & Co., Inc. Publishers.

Hoffman, W. J. 1891. "The Midewiwin or 'Grand Medicine Society' of the Ojibwa." *7th Annual Report of the Bureau of American Ethnology,* pp. 143-300. Washington: Smithsonian Institution.

Hough, T., and W. T. Sedgwick. 1918. *The Human Machine.* Boston: Ginn & Co.

Hutchinson, W. 1922. *A Handbook of Health.* Boston, New York, Chicago, San Francisco: Houghton Mifflin Co.

Jahoda, G. 1975. *The Trail of Tears.* New York: Holt, Rinehart, & Winston Co.

Johnson, C. 1896. *What They Say in New England.* New York: Columbia University Press.

Johnston, H. H. 1910. *The Negro in America.* London: Methuen & Co, Ltd.

Just, A. 1903. *Return to Nature.* New York: The Volunteer Press.

Kellogg, L. P., ed. 1917. *Early Narrations of the Northwest.* New York: Barnes and Noble, Inc.

Kenton, E., ed. 1927. *The Indians of North America.* Volumes 1 & 2. Edited from *The Jesuit Relations and Allied Documents.* 1896. New York: Harcourt, Brace & Co.

Keynes, G., ed. 1951 *The Apologie and Treatise of Ambroise Paré.* London: Falcon Educational Books.

King, L. S. 1958. *The Medical World of the 18th Century.* Chicago: University of Chicago Press.

King, L. S. 1978. *The Philosophy of Medicine.* Cambridge, MA: Harvard University Press.

King, L. S. 1970. *The Road to Medical Enlightenment.* London: MacDonald & Co.

Kowalchik, C., and W. H. Hylton, eds. 1987. *Rodale's Illustrated Encyclopedia of Herbs.* Emmaus, PA: Rodale Press.

Kramer, F. R. 1964. *Voices in the Valley.* Madison, WI: The University of Wisconsin Press.

Kuhns, O. 1901. *The German and Swiss Settlements of Colonial Pennsylvania.* New York: Henry Holt & Co. Publisher.

Lankester, R. 1913. *Science From an Easy Chair*. New York: Henry Holt and Co.

Lapidus, I. M. 1988. *A History of Islamic Societies*. New York & Cambridge, G.B.: Cambridge University Press.

Lorand, A. 1926. *Old Age Deferred*. Philadelphia: F. A. Davis Co. Publisher.

Lust, J. 1970. *The Herb Book*. New York: Bantam Books.

Macfadden, B. 1925. *Headaches--How Caused and How Cured*. New York: Macfadden Publications, Inc.

McGrew, R. E. 1985. *Encyclopedia of Medical History*. New York: McGraw-Hill Book Co.

McGuigan, H. A., and E. K. Krug. 1942. *An Introduction to Materia Medica and Pharmacology*. St. Louis: The C. V. Mosby Co.

McKechnie, J. L., ed. 1983. *Webster's New Universal Unabridged Dictionary*. New York: New World Dictionaries/Simon and Schuster.

____. 1926. *Medical Essays by Medicus*. Editor and printer unknown.

____. 1940. *The Merck Manual of Therapeutics and Materia Medica*. 7th ed. Rahway, NJ: Merck & Co., Inc.

____. 1993. *Merriam-Webster's Medical Dictionary*. Springfield, MA: Merriam-Webster, Inc.

Milburn, W. 1860. *The Pioneers, Preachers, and People of the Mississippi Valley*. New York: Derby and Jackson Press.

Modell, W., and A. Lansing. 1972. *Drugs*. New York: Time Life Books.

Mondat, C.V. 1844. *On Sterility in the Male and Female--Its Causes and Treatment*. New York: J.S. Redfield, Clinton Hall. Boston: Saxton, Peirce, & Co.

Mooney, J. 1892. "The Sacred Formulas of the Cherokees." *7th Annual Report of the Bureau of American Ethnology*, pp. 301-397. Washington: Smithsonian Institution.

___. 1988. *The New Encyclopedia Britannica*. Volumes 8 & 28. Chicago: Encyclopedia Britannica Inc.

Nuland, S. B. 1989. *Doctors--The Biography of Medicine*. New York: Vintage Books.

Osborn, O. T., and M. Fishbein. 1918. *Handbook of Therapy*. Chicago: American Medical Assoc.

Osler, W. 1908. *An Alabama Student and Other Biographical Essays*. London: Oxford University Press.

Pagel, W. 1982. *Joan Baptista Van Helmont*. Cambridge, London: Cambridge University Press.

Palmer, T. 1984. *The Admirable Secrets of Physick and Chyrurgery*. New Haven & London: Yale University Press.

Palos, Stephen. 1971. *The Chinese Art of Healing*. New York: Herder & Herder Co.

Pfeiffer, C. J. 1985. *The Art and Practice of Western Medicine in the Early 19th Century*. Jefferson, NC & London: McFarland and Co., Inc.

Pickard, M. E., and R. C. Buley. 1946. *The Midwest Pioneer*. New York: Henry Schuman Co.

Polley, J., ed. 1978. *American Folklore and Legend*. New York: Reader's Digest Assoc.

___. *Register of Deeds*. 1882-1890. Milwaukee, WI: Milwaukee County Courthouse.

Robinson, V. 1946. *Victory Over Pain*. New York: Henry Schuman, Inc.

Robinson, W. J. 1937. *Medical Sex Dictionary*. New York: Eugenics Publishing Co., Inc.

Roe, E. T. 1903. *Webster's New Standard Dictionary of the English Language*. Chicago: Laird and Lee Publishers.

Roget, P. M. 1992. *Roget's International Thesaurus*. 5th edition. Ed. R. L. Chapman. New York: HarperCollins Publishers.

Rosenberger, J. L. 1923. *The Pennsylvania Germans*. Chicago: The University of Chicago Press.

Rosner, F., and S. Kottek, eds. 1993. *Moses Maimonides--Physician, Scientist, and Philosopher*. Northvale, NJ: Jason Aronson, Inc.

Rossiter, F. M. 1910. *The Practical Guide to Health*. Washington, D.C.: Review and Herald Publishing Assoc.

Rothstein, W. G. 1972. *American Physicians in the Nineteenth Century*. Baltimore: The Johns Hopkins University Press.

Ruddock, E. H. 1926. *Vitalogy*. Chicago: Vitalogy Assoc. Publisher.

Schlissel, L., B. Gibbens, and E. Hampsten. 1989. *Far From Home*. New York: Schocken Books, Inc.

Shryock, R. H. 1936. *The Development of Modern Medicine*. Madison, WI: University of Wisconsin Press.

Shryock, R. H. 1967. *Medical Licensing in America, 1650-1965*. Baltimore, Maryland: The Johns Hopkins Press.

Skeat, W. W. 1993. *The Concise Dictionary of English Etymology*. Hertfordshire, England: Wordsworth Editions, Ltd.

Sonnedecker, G. 1963. *Kremers and Urdang's History of Pharmacy*. 3rd ed. Philadelphia: J.B. Lippincott & Co.

Stedman, T. L. 1942. *Stedman's Shorter Medical Dictionary*. Chicago: American Publishers Corporation.

Stoudt, J. J. 1973. *Sunbonnets and Shoofly Pies*. New York: Castle Books.

Strickland, W. P., ed. 1856. *Autobiography of Peter Cartwright, the Backwoods Preacher*. York: Carlton and Porter Co.

Sweet, W. W., ed. 1916. *Circuit-Rider Days in Indiana*. Indianapolis: W.K. Steward.

Tanner, H. H., ed. 1987. *Atlas of the Great Lakes Indian History*. Norman: University of Oklahoma Press.

Taylor, W. C. 1871. *A Physician's Counsels to Women in Health and Disease*. Springfield, IL: W. J. Holland & Co.

Vogel, V. J. 1970. *American Indian Medicine*. Norman: University of Oklahoma Press.

Weekly, E. 1921. *An Etymological Dictionary of Modern English*. New York: E. P. Dutton & Co.

Wells, S. R. 1889. *New Physiognomy*. New York: Fowler & Wells Co. Publishers.

Weslager, C. A. 1973. *Magic Medicines of the Indians*. Somerset, NJ: The Middle Atlantic Press.

White, T. H. 1978. *In Search of History*. New York: Harper and Row Publishers.

Williams, G. 1975. *The Age of Agony*. London: Constable & Co., Ltd.

Williams, G. 1981, *The Age of Miracles*. Chicago: Academy Publishing Co.

Wilson, C. R., and W. Ferris, eds. 1989. *Encyclopedia of Southern Culture*. Chapel Hill, NC: University of North Carolina Press.

Wissler, C. 1940. *Indians of the United States*. Garden City, NJ: Double Day & Co., Inc.

Wood, G. B., and F. Bache, eds. 1873. *The Dispensatory of the United States of America.* Philadelphia: J.B. Lippincott & Co.

Wood, H. C., Jr., C. H. LaWall, H. H. Youngken, A. Osol, I. Griffith, and L. Gerschenfeld, eds. 1937. *The Dispensatory of the United States of America.* Philadelphia: J.B. Lippincott & Co.

Wright, J. S. 1868. *Chicago: Past, Present, Future.* Chicago: Horton & Leonard Printers.

Wright, R. 1927. *Hawkers and Walkers in Early America.* New York: Frederick Ungar Publishing Co.

Yoder, D. 1990. *Discovering American Folklife.* Ann Arbor: U.M.I. Research Press.